The Royal Swedish Longevity Diet & Weight Control Program

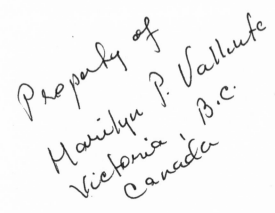

Property of
Marilyn P. Vallute
Victoria, B.C.
Canada

The Royal Swedish Longevity Diet & Weight Control Program

Originally published as *The Royal Swedish Diet & Weight Control Program*

Zina Provendie

with special medical consultant
Dr. Per-Olof Åstrand
and advisor Berit Brattnäs

GROSSET & DUNLAP
A FILMWAYS COMPANY
Publishers • New York

Library of Congress catalog card number: 78-55541

ISBN: 0-448-16186-9

First Grosset & Dunlap printing

Printed in the United States of America

To
Al and Bill
with gratitude for their love
and to the people of Sweden
for the gift of their way of life

EDITORIAL PREPARATION

Design
Susan Lusk

Assistant
Denise Weber

Photography
Frank Lusk

Sports Advisor
William Behrensen

Editors
David Sachs
Dorothy Chamberlain

Models
Doreen Lusk
William Behrensen

Typesetting
Scarlett Letters

ACKNOWLEDGEMENTS

I am very grateful to Berit Bratt-näs, former Director of the Swedish Sports Foundation, for her generous help in authenticating the information in this manuscript, and to Dr. Per-Olof Astrand, who was willing to take time from a busy practice in Sweden to act as special medical consultant for this work. To the Swedish Consulate General in New York, and in particular to Eva Von Uslar, of the Swedish Information Service, my gratitude for help in obtaining photographs of the famous Swedish Sofia girls and the Idla girls in action.

CONTENTS

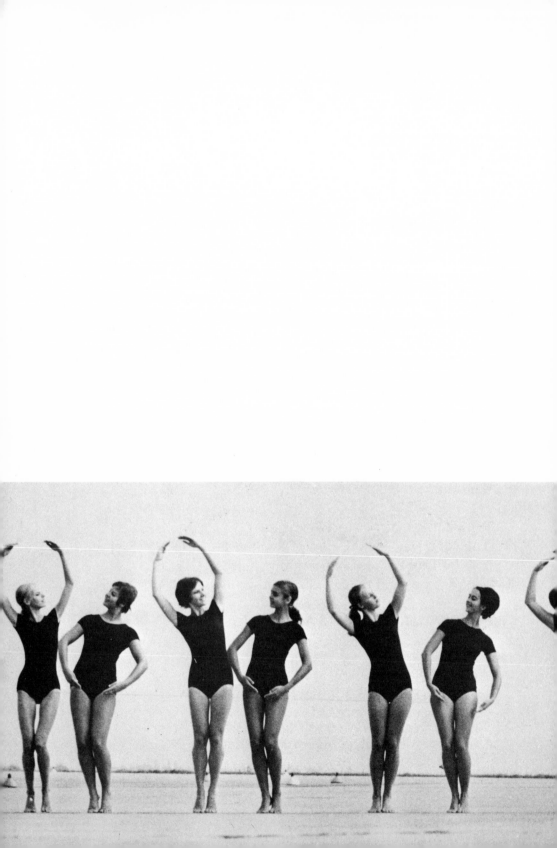

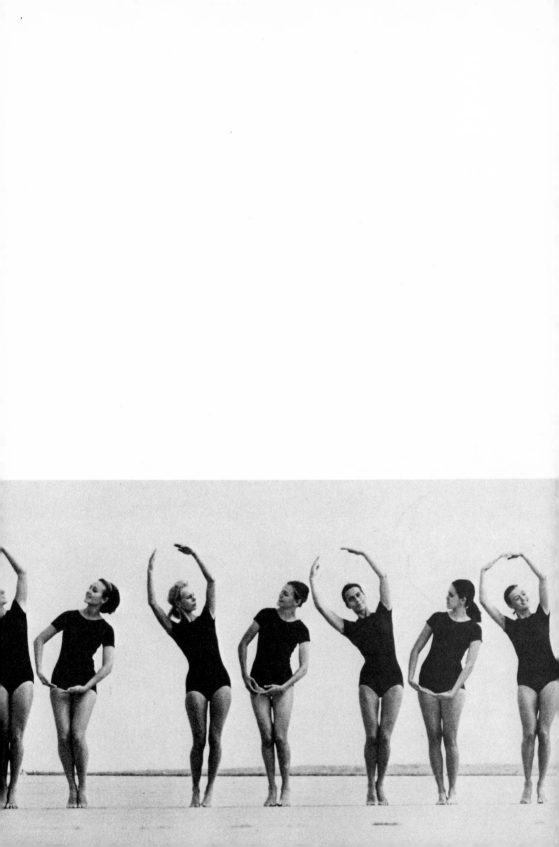

The Royal Swedish Longevity Diet & Weight Control Program

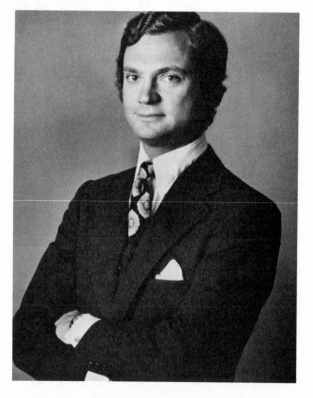

Carl XVI Gustaf, the new king of Sweden, heads a nation that has made beauty and radiant good health building blocks for a joyous way of life.

INTRODUCTION

Think of Scotland and you envision kilts and bagpipes. Ireland? Shamrocks and the Blarney Stone. Holland? Windmills and tulips.

But think of Sweden and the image is handsome, blond Vikings, men and women radiating good health and a special joy in living.

"The sea or mountain air has blown through them for so many centuries that their lungs, too, are washed," Marya Mannes wrote.* "To see men without the greenish pallor or larded white of our own city workers, to see girls with unfussed hair and uncaked skin, the blood near the surface of unlipsticked mouths, is to rediscover a lost beauty."

Share in that rediscovery. Make that beauty, that good health, that pride in your person truly yours through the exercises, nutritional guidance and counsel in *The Royal Swedish Longevity Diet & Weight Control Program.*

These precepts were physical fitness rules that allowed the late King Gustaf VI Adolf to live an extraordinarily active life for more than 90 years. Until his death, the late king went to Rome every year for archaeological digs before his summer retreat to the palace at Sofiero—where he worked in the garden. His favorite hobbies were archaeology and gardening. The same physical and mental health

* *As quoted in **The Scandinavians** by Donald S. Connery, Simon and Schuster, New York, 1966.*

habits guided his father, King Gustaf V, who played a great game of tennis until his death at 92. The new King of Sweden, handsome young Carl XVI Gustaf, follows in his father's and grandfather's footsteps.

The Royal Swedish way of keeping fit is a way of life not only for the royal family, but for all Swedes, from typist to storekeeper to homemaker. In it you will discover a full mental and physical health program that will improve your self-image and also the way others see you. You will stand taller, straighter, with a posture showing confidence and vitality. And the gymnastics program that helps you achieve it is exhilarating and fun.

Eating will no longer be accompanied by sighs of miserable resignation. The Swedish diet way to enjoyable, nonfattening gourmet

Right: The easy rhythm of a well-mastered group exercise is demonstrated by another famous physical culture group, Swedish housewives, officeworkers, students, and professional people who are students of Ernst Idla.

Below: Sweden's famous Sofia Girls stage a display of wand exercises in front of the Town Hall in Stockholm, Sweden. Organized some years ago by a brilliant Swedish teacher of physical education, Maja Carlquist, the Sofia girls draw members from all ages and categories, and prove that everyone can be beautiful.

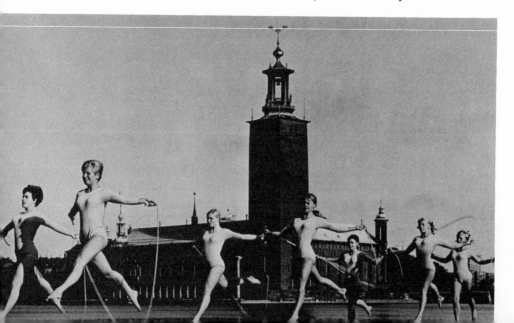

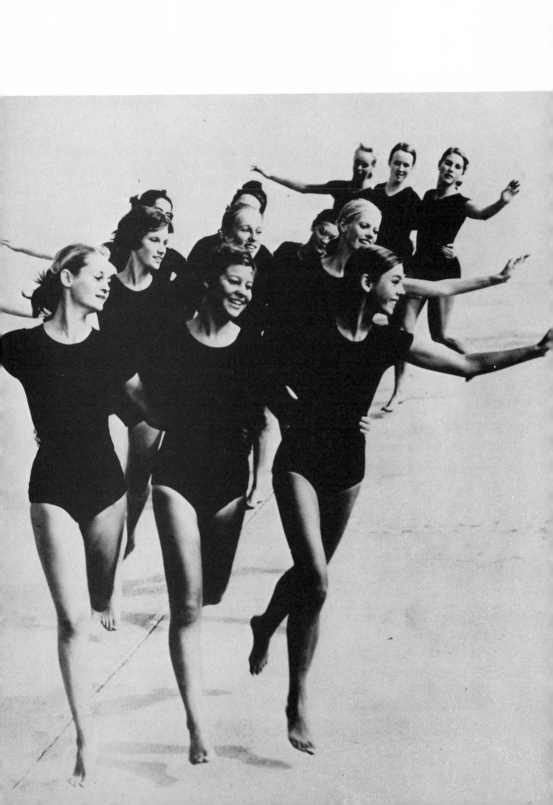

dishes will delight you. It includes recipes you can share without guilt or scale-facing remorse.

You will become familiar with herbal recipes for health and hygiene and home spa mixtures, recipes that have been used for more than 300 years.

One by one, you will translate your goals to achievements: serenity, contentment, strength, personal pride, a mental attitude of health and optimism, a positive physical presence and the joy of being able to say, "I like the way I look. I like the way I think. I like me!"

Proper exercise makes proper eating easier: proper exercise and proper diet together are crucial factors in the new holistic approach to health and long life. Holistic medicine says strengthen the whole body through proper exercise and diet and mental outlook, and many undiagnosed illnesses will clear up of their own accord.

Dr. Lee Steiner, Ph.D., now past sixty and a practicing psychologist with an active clientele in the world's toughest city, New York, walks like a girl, thinks like a young woman, and carries the full load of a mature doctor. She says:

> To live a long and vigorous and joyful life, write exercise into your daily living, just as you include combing your hair or bathing. There has to be time for it, a routine for it. Begin slowly, don't overdo. Work up a routine and make it regular. And enjoy it! Enjoying your exercises is important! A happy exercise routine can help control the stresses that cause killer emotions. (See The Longevity Test that begins page 249.) Dr. Steiner recommends the avoidance of overindulgence as well. "Too much alcohol, too much smoking, too much eating—these waste and overload the system.

How much is too much? Anything that leaves you exhausted, uncomfortable.

How much exercise is needed to improve longevity? Enough to stir you up, get you panting a little, get the blood going. One of the consequences of aging is the loss of the ability of cells to reproduce. When cells stop reproducing, we start to atrophy. To counteract this, we must make sure that healthy blood is feeding every cell in the body, especially the brain and nervous system.

That old saying "Use it or lose it!" applies to life, too!

PART I
BEFORE YOU BEGIN

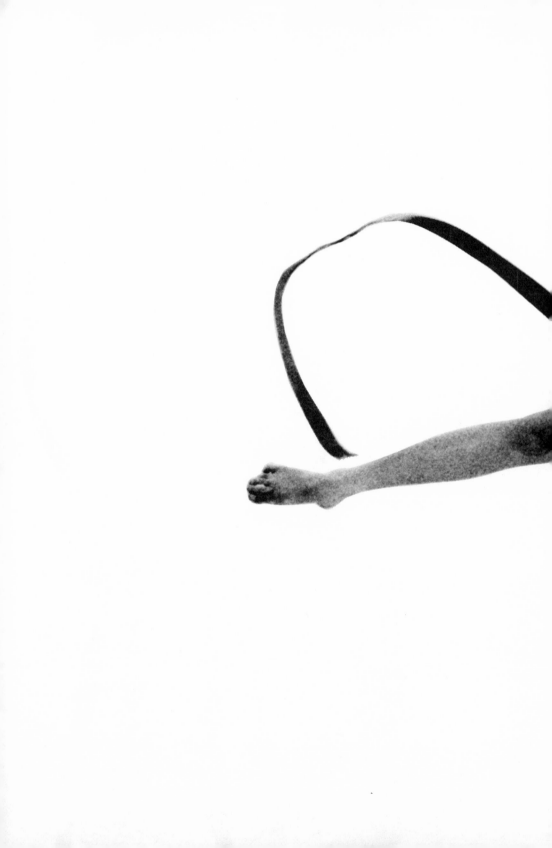

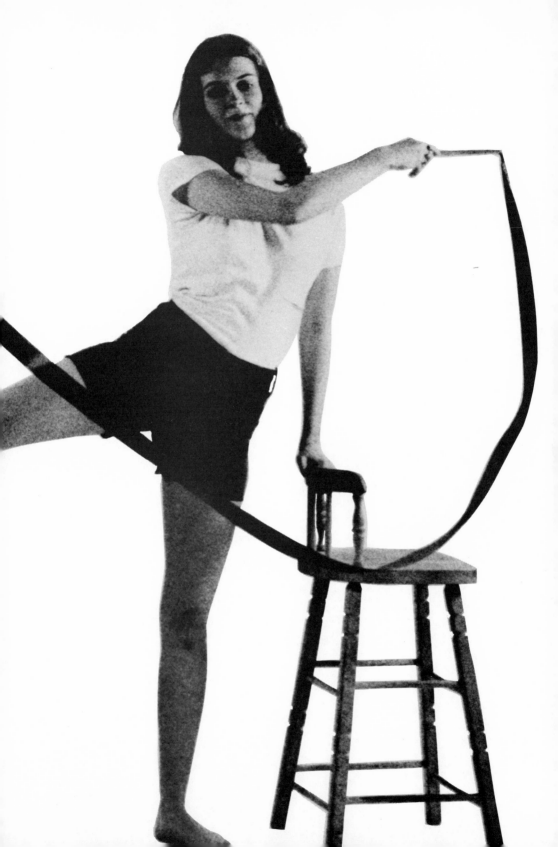

ONE

CHARTING YOUR GOALS

Before you begin the Royal Swedish program, chart your goals. No one need tell you whether you should be thinner or fatter. The reflection in your mirror will tell you all you need to know. Nor can any single chart dictate how many pounds should be shed or gained. No two persons were ever cast in exactly the same mold. You are—and should always recognize yourself as—a unique individual.

If you are exceptionally large boned, you may always weigh more than many charts say you should. The chart below is a guide only. Trust your own eye and judgment. Excessive dieting may give you a lean and haggard look, which won't compliment you at all. Inspect your figure objectively. If you can pinch yourself at the waist and inner thighs and come up with an inch or more of fatty padding, yes, you are overweight.

YOUR WEIGHT-BY-HEIGHT GOAL

Skeletal Frame	Weight Base	Weight Goal
Women: Small Men: Small	95 pounds 100 pounds	Both men and women should add
Women: Medium Men: Medium	100 pounds 110 pounds	five pounds to the Weight Base for every
Women: Large Men: Large	105 pounds 115 pounds	inch of height over five feet.

These figures may safely vary plus or minus six pounds.

To resolve the dilemma of the number of inches you wish to trim away, use a wrist "calculator": Determine your body-measurement goals by the circumference of your wrist. First measure your wrist with a flexible measuring tape. Then take these measurements:

- The waist below the rib cage.
- The hips at the fullest part of the buttocks.
- The thighs halfway between the knee and the groin.
- The calves around the fullest part, a little below the knee.
- The ankle just above the anklebone.

Ideally, your waist should equal four and a quarter times the circumference of your wrist. Your hips, six times your wrist; the thighs, three and a half times; the calves, two and a quarter times; your ankles, one and a half times.

Your weight *will* fluctuate from day to day. Keep tabs on the reasons for these weight changes and then you will be able to control them. *When* your weight increased and *what* you ate on that particular day will give you the *why*. You will find, for example, that a holiday feast or celebration will give you the answer to your mysterious weight gain.

Duplicate these sample record sheets in a notebook or a month-at-a-glance diary, and keep it near your weight scale.

MONTH: _____

Sunday	Monday	Tuesday	Wednesday	Thursday	Friday	Saturday

DAY-BY-DAY FOOD INTAKE

	Sun.	Mon.	Tues.	Wed.	Thurs.	Fri.	Sat.
Breakfast							
Lunch							
Dinner							
Snacks							

THE BODY LANGUAGE OF POSTURE

You need never say a word to anyone about the kind of person you are. Your posture will say it for you. The way you carry yourself is the first clue to the opinion you have of yourself and the impression you make on others.

A slovenly, S-shape silhouette, with lowered head, sunken chest, and protruding abdomen, has its own body language: the droop of apology, a disintegrating self-esteem, and a loss in the joy of living.

You don't need a crown to help you walk regally. But a royal bearing isn't possible unless you put your bones in alignment.

Wear nothing or next to nothing. Take a long look at yourself, preferably in a three-way mirror.

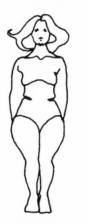
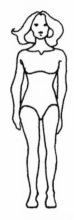

Do you look like this?   You should look like this!

• Find your center. This isn't mysterious or metaphysical. Your body has a natural center, which extends from the pelvis to the base of the skull—your spine. That spine, the body's center, must support your whole torso.

• Gravity is the enemy of maturity. With age, gravity pulls everything downward. The word to remember is LIFT!

1. Start with the crown of your head, as though it were being lifted from your neck by an invisible force pulling at your head's very top.

2. Imagine two firm but loving hands holding your head over each ear and lifting your head up, up out of your neck.

3. Lift your chin so that it is exactly parallel with the floor. Now, with your head up, look straight out at the world. Unflinching. Proudly.

4. Press your shoulder blades down, giving a long line to the neck. A long, straight neck gives grace to women, strength to men. Your shoulders should be in their natural position; don't force them back. This would merely tip the head forward.

5. Lift your chest without lifting the shoulders. Give your lungs room to function! Lifting the chest high will not only let your lungs fill freely but will also counteract the impression of withdrawal conveyed by the sunken-chest posture. (ASIDE TO WOMEN: Carrying the chest high will also help strengthen those fragile bands of tissue that support the breasts and thus will prevent the sag of gravity.)

6. Lift your rib cage out of your waist, and tighten the abdominal muscles. Here is Swedish magic from the mountain trolls! You will instantly whittle an inch off your waistline and gain an inch in height!

7. Tip the pelvis forward by tucking your buttocks under, lifting the stomach so that you can

8. Flatten the small of your back against a wall.

9. Relax your arms at your sides, and "release" the elbows. Avoid locked, stiff elbows.

10. If your hands hang stiffly, "shake" them out, and then let them hang naturally. The natural position for the fingers is to let them curl and not to extend them stiffly. Let the hands brush lightly against the legs. Avoid "hanging out the wrists to dry" by extending them even an inch from your sides.

11. Turn and face the mirror. If your legs seem to be bowed, or if there is a space between your calves, this bowlegged appearance can be cured isometrically—unless the bone structure in your legs is curved.
    a. Contract your calf muscles by pulling the calves together until they touch. Hold this position for ten counts, and *Se dar!* (*Voila!* in Swedish)
    b. Release your calf muscles slowly. Do not release with muscle tension.
    c. Repeat at various times during the day, whenever you are standing.
        Keep the bowlegged look from reappearing by wearing shoes with even support, and never wear shoes with run-down heels.

12. Hold your body erect, with the small of your back flattened and your weight carried forward over the balls of your feet, so that your heels feel free, even though they are resting on the floor.

13. Double-check the small of your back. Is it still touching the wall? If it is not, here's an exercise that will help you sustain the straight-back posture.
    a. Facing into the room, step nine inches away from the wall.
    b. Flex your knees slightly, and rest your buttocks against the wall.

    c.   Bend at the waist, and drop forward limply. Let your arms dangle loosely.

    d.   Unroll slowly. Let each vertebra touch the wall gently, and straighten your knees slowly as you step closer to the wall and slide up against it, so that each vertebra in your upper back touches the wall.

YOUR WALK

Rehearse your walk in stocking feet or barefoot.
Head up,
Chin lifted, parallel to the floor,
Chest high, with rib cage pulled up out of the waist,
Back stretched long and straight, with pelvis tipped under,
Abdomen pulled in, breathe normally as you release your knees and lift your left heel off the floor to bring your body weight forward as you
Step forward with your right foot, swinging your leg from the hip joint.
When your weight is firmly on your right foot,
Step forward with your left foot, lifting the right heel to transfer weight smoothly from right to left.
NOTE: Let your arms swing freely, but correctly. The left arm should swing forward as you step out with the right foot, simultaneously swinging the right arm back: right foot forward, left arm forward, right arm back, left foot forward, right arm forward, and so on.
Keep knees released, not bent. Locking the knees rigidly would give your walk a jerky stride.
When walking—
• Do not place one foot directly in front of the other. This would give your walk a sway and throw your hips from side to side.
• Toe out very slightly to retain balance.
• The length of your stride should be not less than the length of your foot. Short steps would make your walk choppy.
• Keep a space of about three inches between your feet.

YOUR SEATED POSTURE

Let the back of your leg tell you where a chair is.

Lower yourself into a chair without aiming for it with your bottom.

Sit into a chair, not on the edge.

Keep your rib cage lifted even when you lounge. It is possible to sit comfortably without squashing yourself accordion fashion.

Walk, sit, or stand purposefully, not tentatively; proudly, not apologetically.

Whether or not others get a favorable impression from the way you stand, sit, or move isn't half as important as the reality that attaining good posture is your first step toward being physically fit to live and to live longer and happier.

PART II
GETTING STARTED

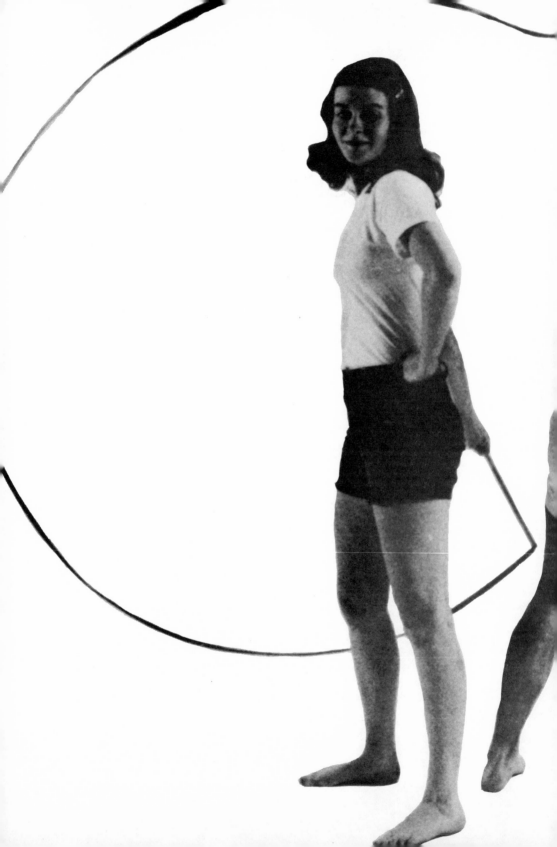

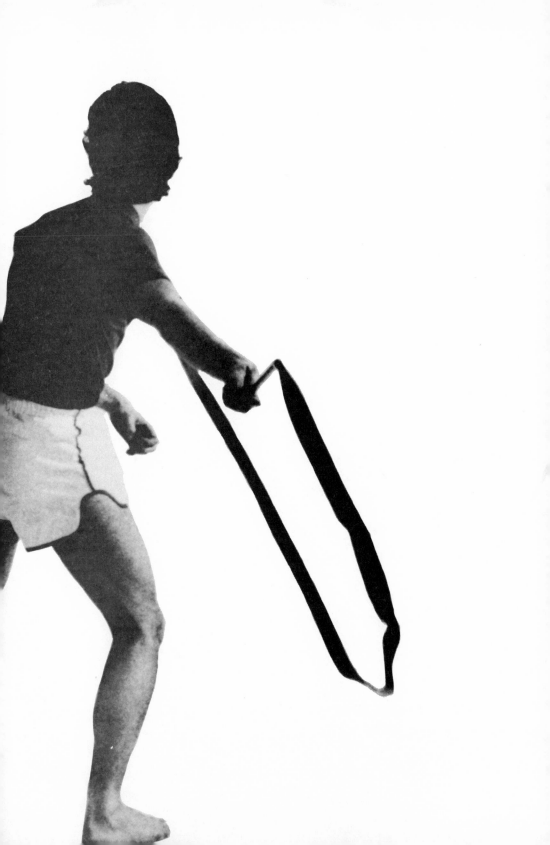

TWO

SWEDISH
LIMBER-UP EXERCISES

The Royal Swedish Physical-Fitness Programs are specifically structured to involve the exercising of every major muscle group in the body. Each program is designed to fill many needs, whatever your age, sex, physical condition, or personal requirement.

Warm-up with the Basic Limbering Program before performing the rest of your slim-down routine. Muscles that are "warmed" are more pliant, and they will not cramp or strain. Even if you have time only to go through your Limbering sequences or those exercises in a special category (i.e., Office Exercises, Fitness for Housewives, Exercises for Sports, etc.), you will discover that they will help you be more supple and physically alert. Your circulation will be improved. You will tire less frequently. Tension will dissolve, and you will be able to perform your daily activities with considerably less stress and strain.

THE ROYAL SWEDISH MAGIC WAND

Exercise programs are usually offered temptingly packaged and tied with promises. If intelligently followed, they often will produce improved muscle tone and a trimmer figure. But fitness routines can degenerate into a series of dull contortions. The Swedish wand exercises, done to music, make it all interesting and fun. Keeping those ribbons going is a challenge you will really enjoy.

The Royal Swedish Magic Wand Exercises and free-play routines, if instituted as part of your everyday activity, can help with rapid weight-loss, and will awaken and revitalize sluggish circulation, strengthen your heart, and thereby increase your chances at a longer lifespan. And, in a unique way, your magic wand will, through its graceful visual patterns and musical accompaniment, put you in closer touch with your body's natural rhythms and the way you were intended to move. Your Magic Wand Exercise program, with its unusual stress on inventiveness, natural grace, and mobility, will take exercise beyond tedium and make your movements a discovery and a joy.

YOUR MAGIC WAND AND HOW TO USE IT

To make a wand like the one we have used in the photos in this book, staple, tack, or tie a ribbon two inches wide by 12 feet long to a 12- to 14-inch-long wooden ruler, dowel, or small straight stick. Improvise the many varying forms your ribboned wand can make!

From Circles

to Spirals

to Half-Circles

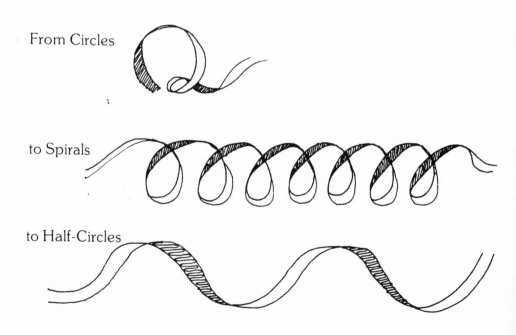

to Arcs

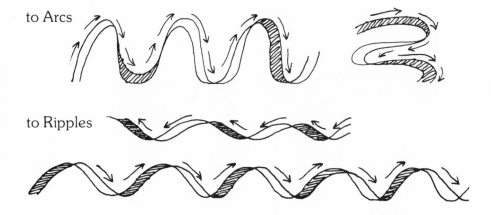

to Ripples

to Vertical Zigs

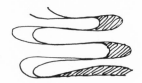

to Horizontal Zags

to Ocean Waves

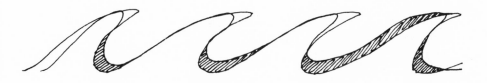

to Mountain Peaks

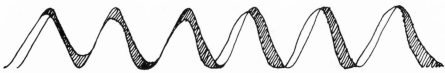

to Figure Eights

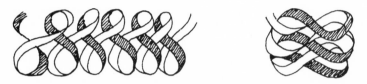

to Letters of the Alphabet.

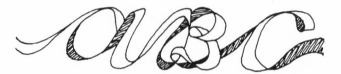

If the music you select becomes louder or faster, you will want to make your arm and wrist movements faster and stronger and vary even more the shapes and sizes of your patterns.

Use your wrist to whip the ribbons into sudden changes of direction and for smaller patterns. Use the varying shapes as an opportunity to stretch! Your wand will inspire you to stretch from ankle to thigh, from thigh to waist, from waist to neck, from neck to the top of your head and to the very ends of your fingertips.

A RULE OF CAUTION:

Do not strain. Your body can actually be hurt by overexertion. Let time and consistency of these pleasurable exercises gradually increase your capacity to perform them—comfortably!

THE MAGIC-WAND GESTURES

The effectiveness of every exercise program stems from the total involvement of all muscles and joints, particularly those frequently neglected, such as shoulder sockets, elbows, wrists, hands, hips, and ankles. Rehearse each wand gesture separately, so that you are certain of getting the physical benefits in each movement. You will also be amazed at your ability to acquire a litheness and grace you thought belonged only to dancers.

The magic of your wand is in its use. Become as familiar with all that it can do as you are with a pen or pencil.

HOW TO HOLD YOUR WAND

Hold your wand as you would a large paintbrush, with the thumb clasping the handle on one side and the four fingers on the other.

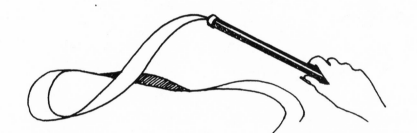

If both hands will be holding the wand, take hold of it as if to hold it in one hand; then place the other hand above it.

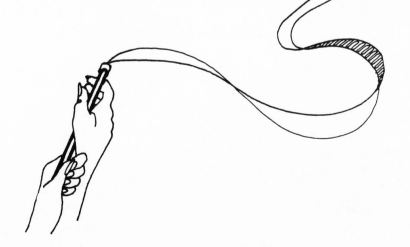

WAND POSITIONS FOR ARMS AND ELBOWS

The rounded elbow is released and lightly flexed.

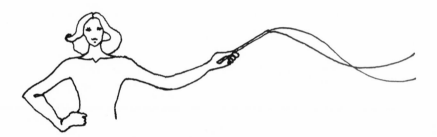

The locked elbow is rigidly straightened.

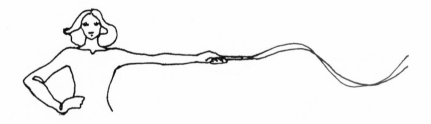

The bent elbow is fully flexed.

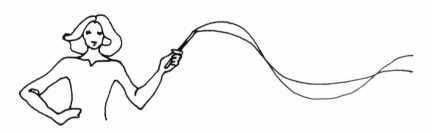

Keep elbows in wand exercises soft and rounded, so the arm will be free to move gracefully, up or down, forward or back, or from right to left and back again.

Avoid locked or bent elbows unless specified by the exercise sequence. The locked- and bent-elbow positions inhibit smooth arm movements and cannot flow into free and graceful patterns.

LET YOUR WRISTS LEAD YOU

And your arms will follow! The variations of the following horizontal, vertical, and curved wand swirls start with the eight wrist-lead positions:

1. Lead with the inner wrist, curving the hand outward, swirling the wand toward the body.

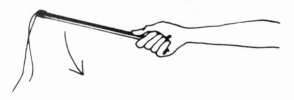

2. Lead with inner wrist, curving hand outward, to swirl wand away from body.

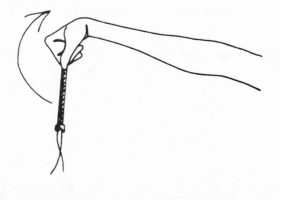

3. Lead with outer wrist; curve hand inward, to swirl wand toward body.

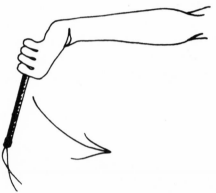

4. Lead with outer wrist; curve hand inward, to swirl wand away from body.

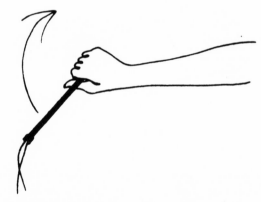

5. Lead with thumb side of the wrist, hand parallel to the floor, palm down, to swirl wand toward the body.

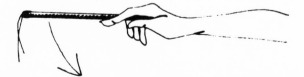

6. Lead with thumb side of wrist, hand parallel to the floor, palm up, to swirl wand away from body.

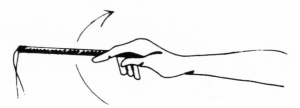

7. Lead with the littlest-finger side of the wrist, hand parallel to the floor, palm up, to swirl wand toward body.

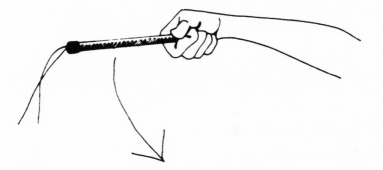

8. Lead with the littlest-finger side of wrist, hand parallel to the floor, palm down, to swirl wand away from the body.

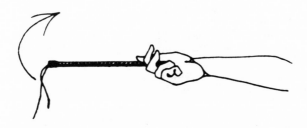

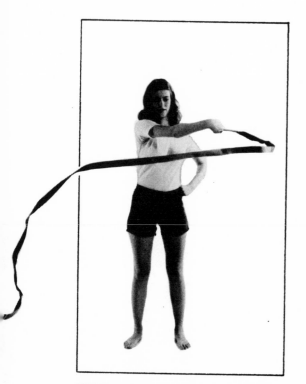

HORIZONTAL WAND SWIRLS

Horizontal Variation No. 1

START:
Wand in right hand, raise right arm to the side, shoulder level; left hand on hip.
1. Curve hand outward. Lead with inner wrist as you swirl wand across body, shoulder level.
2. When right hand is opposite left shoulder, curve hand inward, and lead with the back of the wrist as you return right arm to starting position.
3. Continue swirling wand horizontally left and right across your body in rhythmic sequence.
4. Repeat entire variation, 1 through 3, with left hand.

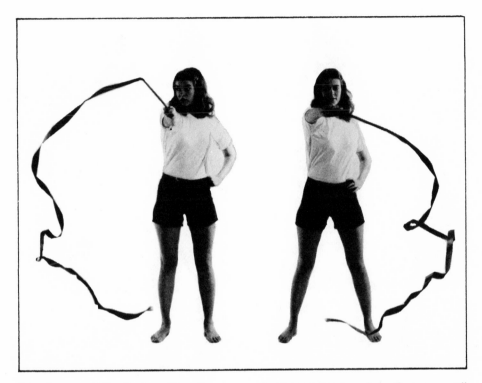

Horizontal Variation No. 2

START:
Hold wand in right hand, arm raised shoulder level; left hand on hip.
1. Curving hand outward, lead with the inner wrist as you swirl wand across body from right to left; then

2. Turn your hand so that you still lead with the inner wrist, now swirling from left to right. Continue sequence several times.
NOTE:
This variation is identical with Variation 1, except that the hand turns at a change in direction, so that you constantly lead with the inner wrist, curving the hand outward. Follow this procedure whether the direction is from right to left, or left to right.
3. Repeat entire sequence, 1 and 2, with left hand.

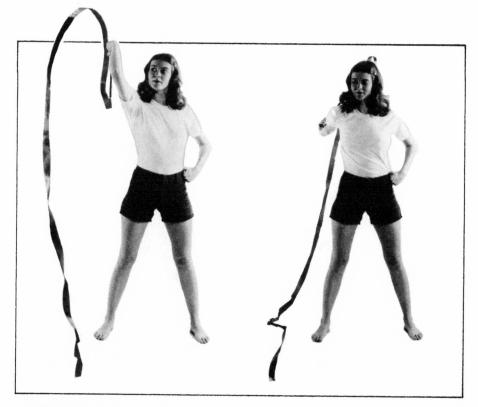

VERTICAL WAND SWIRLS

Vertical Variation No. 1

START:
Holding wand in either hand, raise arm to the side, heel of hand parallel to the floor.
1. With hands curved back, lead with inner wrist as you swirl wand downward, then

2. Turn hand, and still leading with the inner wrist, swirl wand upward at the side. Continue swirling wand up and down several times. Then swirl wand in front of you, vertically, and then behind you.

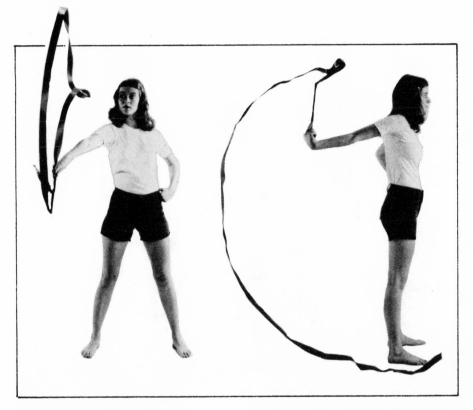

Vertical Variation No. 2

START:
With a wand in right hand, raise arm
to the side, heel of hand parallel to the
floor.
1. Lead with inner wrist to swirl wand
downward, then

2. Do not turn hand as in Vertical
Variation 1, but lead with the back of
the wrist, hand curved inward, to swirl
wand up and continue sequence 1
and 2 several times. Gradually twist at
the waist, turning right, and continue
to swirl wand in a vertical zig-zag
pattern.

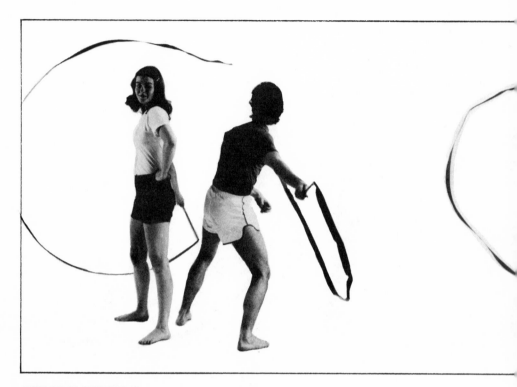

CIRCLE SWIRLS

Use rotating wrist movements for
small circles. Use full arm and shoulder socket for large circles, turning the
hand in changing from downward to
upward wand swirls.

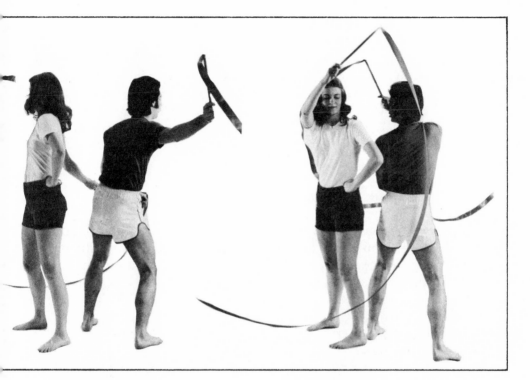

SPIRAL SWIRLS

Use technique for Circle Swirls, but stretch circles into spirals by elongating the circular movements.

ARC SWIRLS

Use full arm and shoulder, changing wrist movements and turning the hand to accommodate the varying sizes and directions of arc shapes.

YOUR CALISTHENIC WARDROBE

If you are in your office, kick off your shoes, and remove inhibiting coat or jacket, watch, jewelry, and belt (at the risk of falling trousers).

But if you are in the privacy of your own home, exercise in any garment that gives you room to move and that will stretch as you do. A leotard, if well cut, is excellent; or you can improvise by wearing shorts, an elasticized bathing suit, or nothing at all.

PERSONALIZE YOUR EXERCISE PROGRAM

• Exercise to music! Let your emotional response to melody add to your enjoyment of your exercises. Tune in your favorite radio musical program or use records. Tangos, fox trots, folk songs—Swedish men and women exercise to any type of music the mood of the moment may inspire, be it a polka, a waltz, or a schottische, musical comedy tunes, jazz, or Mozart's country dances.
• Wake up to music, and start each day with a cat stretch. Feel the stretch—in your back, your arms, your legs.
• Inhale and exhale deeply and evenly while you're exercising. The oxygen you breathe into the bloodstream will help repair and renew all your body cells and carry away toxic wastes.
• At various intervals throughout the day, here is a miraculous routine to add to your height, shrink the waistline, and tighten abdomen muscles: Lift the rib cage, contract the abdominal muscles, and hold the muscular contraction for ten counts; then relax slowly. Breathe naturally throughout.
• If you are past 40, avoid excessive stretches, very deep knee bends, and jerky movements, particularly with any back exercises.
• Whatever your age, all exercises involving the spine and the knees should be performed carefully and effortlessly, never forced. The vertebrae and the kneecaps are the only parts of the body that do not renew themselves!
• Never do an exercise that is painful. Exercise should help, not hurt. If any single exercise causes pain or even discomfort, it is not for you.

- Move to live. Your regular total body movement will reactivate your whole circulatory system and retard the aging process.
- Note exercises marked with asterisks:
  *Exercises marked with one asterisk are particularly recommended for posture.
  * *Exercises marked with two asterisks are especially effective for the easing of tension and fatigue.
* * *Exercises marked with three asterisks are singularly potent when improvised with a wand. Mix-and-match these sequences with your Magic Wand routines in Chapter III.

YOUR DAILY LIMBERING SERIES

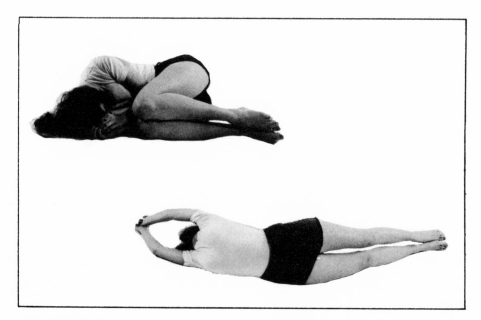

CAT STRETCH

GOALS:
To limber and stretch whole body.

START:
Lie down on bed or floor, curled up, on your side. Make yourself as compact as possible.

1. Slowly uncurl; stretch out, straightening legs and stretching arms above your head. Then roll over to the other side and curl back up, arms around knees, to starting position. Repeat entire sequence, curling up on each side, six times.

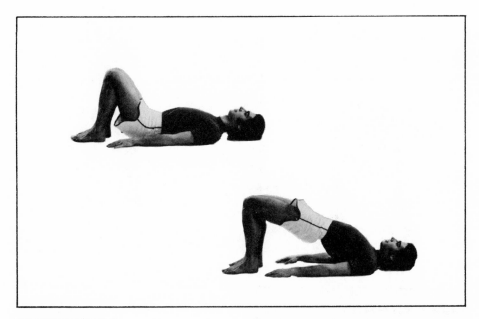

TRUNK LIFT *

GOALS:
To limber back muscle, and tighten and tone abdomen and buttocks.
START:
Lie flat on floor with legs approximately 12 inches apart, arms at sides.
1. Bring knees up to bent knee position, with feet flat on floor.

2. Contract buttock muscles, and slowly a) lift buttocks from floor; then b) lift small of back from floor; then c) lift upper part of back, and hold complete lift for five counts. Relax slowly, lowering a) first, upper back, then b) small of back, and finally, c) lower buttocks to the floor, and rest in starting position for ten seconds. Repeat entire sequence three times.

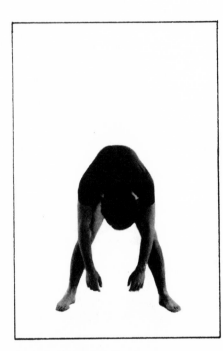 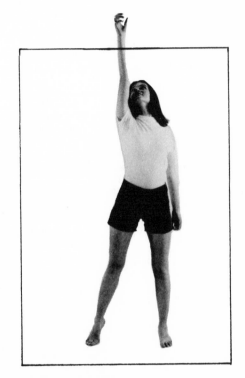

BOW AND STRETCH *

GOALS:
To stretch and limber knees and back, release tension, and improve posture.

START:
Stand; feet shoulders' width apart, arms relaxed at sides.
1. Inhale. As you exhale, flop forward from the waist, letting your head hang loose. Hold for five counts, while continuing to breathe regularly. Gradually straighten knees, then straighten up, one vertebra at a time, until you stand erect.
NOTE:
Do not let your head get ahead of the rest of your spine while you are straightening to erect posture.

ROPE CLIMB * * *

GOALS:
To stretch rib cage and firm up loosely fleshed arms, while circumventing fatigue and tension.

START:
Stand with feet about 20 inches apart, back very straight and chin level.
1. Raise both arms as high as you can, and grasp for the ceiling with first the right hand and then the left hand. (Feel the stretch in your side and rib cage as you reach. The rib cage should be lifted up and out of your waist.) When you have reached as high as you possibly can, comfortably, clench your fist as if to grab a rope; use a pulling motion to pull yourself up, and continue "climbing" rope, alternating right and left reaches, until you have completed ten pull-up movements. Then return to starting position and relax.

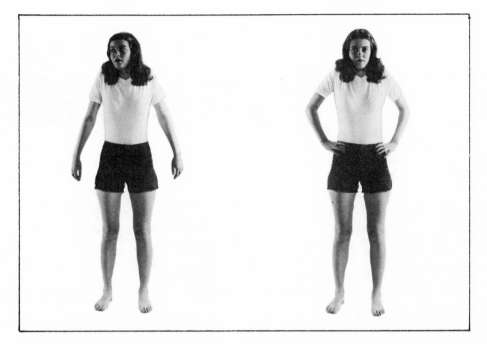

SHOULDER SHRUGS * * *

GOALS:
To stretch and limber shoulders, trimming down dowager (cellulite) pads.

START:
Stand, or sit erectly, back straight and chin level, arms relaxed at your sides.
1. Lift shoulders as high as you can; then lower them. Repeat three times.

2. Rotate right shoulder blade three times clockwise, then three times counterclockwise. Repeat sequence 2 with left shoulder blade; then
3. Rotate both shoulder blades forward three times, back down-and-up three times. Repeat shoulder lift 1 three times, and return to starting position.

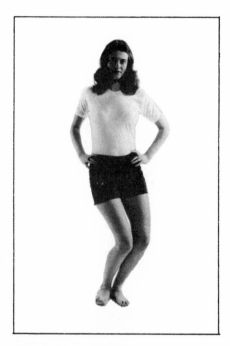

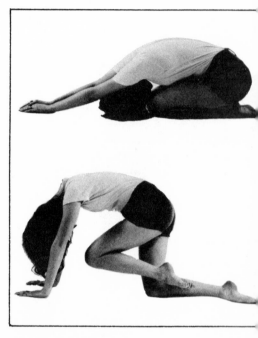

SLALOM TWIST * * *

GOALS:
To limber foot elasticity and upgrade circulation.

START:
Stand, feet three inches apart; raise arms to the sides, just below shoulder level, elbows slightly rounded.
1. Bend knees slightly, and hop on both feet, turning from side to side, twisting from the waist.
NOTE:
Try to keep heels down and to bend your knees as much as you can for each hop.

BACK STRETCH

GOALS:
To stretch and limber back muscles and trim thighs.

START:
On the floor, on your hands and knees.
1. Keep hands on the floor as you rock back on your heels and touch your head to your knees twice. Rise, still on knees, but with arms straightened, with your weight on the heels of your hands and your knees.
2. Keep back straight as you drop your head and lift your right knee up toward your chin, then

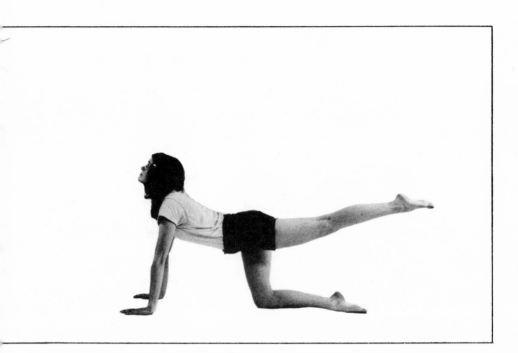

3. Arch your back as your lift your head and stretch your right leg back and up. Repeat sequence twice, then return to starting position and repeat *entire exercise four times. Turn over on your back and rest twenty seconds.*

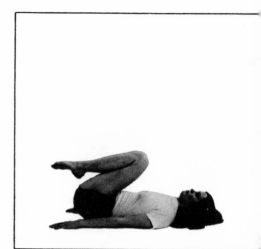

FRONT LEG LIFT *

GOALS:
To maintain leg muscle tone and beautiful posture.

START:
Lie on the floor, legs about six inches apart, arms relaxed at sides.
1. Contract abdominal muscles, and press lower back against floor. Then draw knees up to chest.

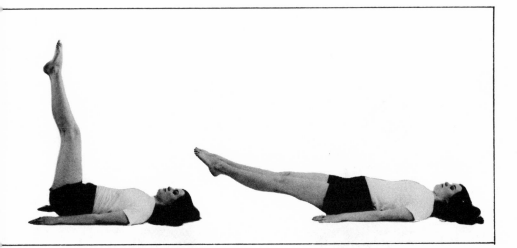

2. Lift both legs, straighten knees, and raise legs. Point toes at ceilings. Hold, and bend both knees, draw them back to chest, as in 1. Then

3. Straighten legs so they are about four inches from the floor, and lower them slowly, returning to starting position. Rest ten seconds, and repeat entire exercise six times.

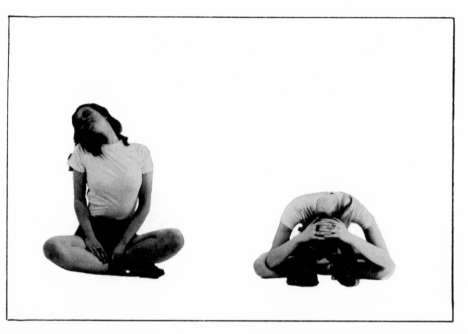

NECK LOOSENERS

GOALS:
To loosen tension in the neck and shoulders.

START:
Sit tailor fashion with arms relaxed, hands in your lap. Let chin and head drop loosely forward.
1. With chin toward right shoulder, roll your head lazily from one side to the other in large semicircles, four times; then

2. Reach up, knit fingers loosely behind you, and without effort, slowly bend forward and touch your forehead to the floor in front. Rest quietly, thinking of tall trees, mountains, and lakes. After 30 seconds, slowly rise to seated position, and repeat entire sequence six times.

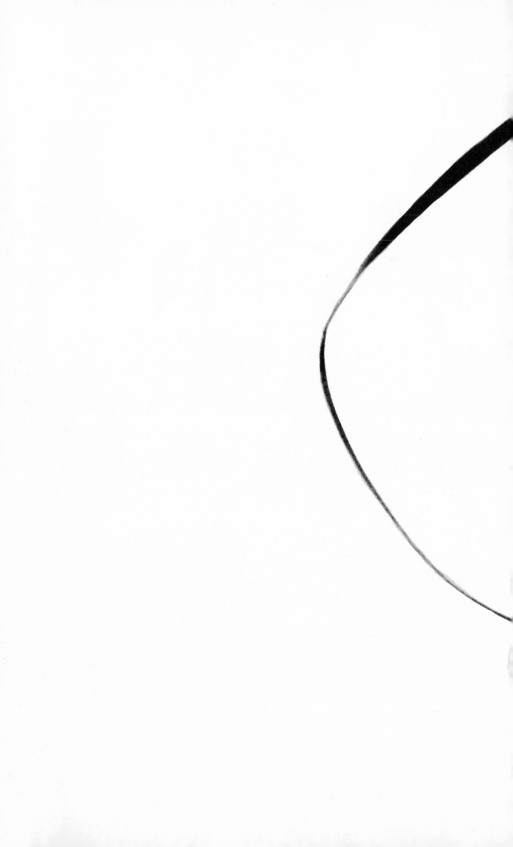

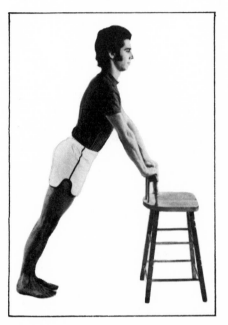

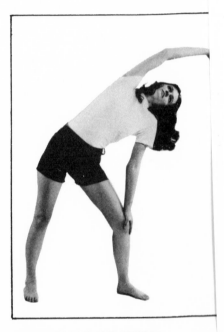

CALVES

GOALS:
To stretch muscles of calves, preventing muscle cramps and tightness.

START:
Stand three feet from wall; keep body straight.
1. Lean forward against wall or a high-backed chair, using your palms against the wall for support. Keep your heels on the floor. Continue to lean until you feel the stretch and pull in the calves. Hold for ten seconds, and return to starting position. Repeat sequence five times.

SIDE SPINE FLEXOR

GOALS:
To stregthen side flexing of spine (while slimming waist and thighs).

START:
Stand legs wide apart, arms extended at sides, shoulder level.
1. Leading with the wrist, swing right arm above head, arching upper torso with the upswing of the arm. Bend knee slightly. Your right palm should be facing up, your left arm lowered to the front of your right thigh. Bounce gently to the left, three times, and slowly return to starting position. Then, repeat raising left arm and bending to the right. Return to starting position, and repeat entire sequence five times.

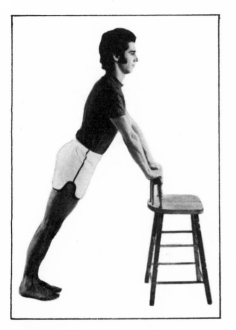 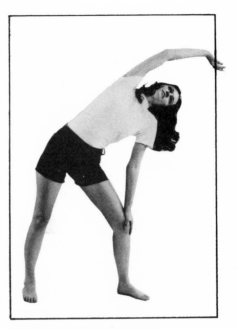

CALVES

GOALS:
To stretch muscles of calves, preventing muscle cramps and tightness.

START:
Stand three feet from wall; keep body straight.
1. Lean forward against wall or a high-backed chair, using your palms against the wall for support. Keep your heels on the floor. Continue to lean until you feel the stretch and pull in the calves. Hold for ten seconds, and return to starting position. Repeat sequence five times.

SIDE SPINE FLEXOR

GOALS:
To stregthen side flexing of spine (while slimming waist and thighs).

START:
Stand legs wide apart, arms extended at sides, shoulder level.
1. Leading with the wrist, swing right arm above head, arching upper torso with the upswing of the arm. Bend knee slightly. Your right palm should be facing up, your left arm lowered to the front of your right thigh. Bounce gently to the left, three times, and slowly return to starting position. Then, repeat raising left arm and bending to the right. Return to starting position, and repeat entire sequence five times.

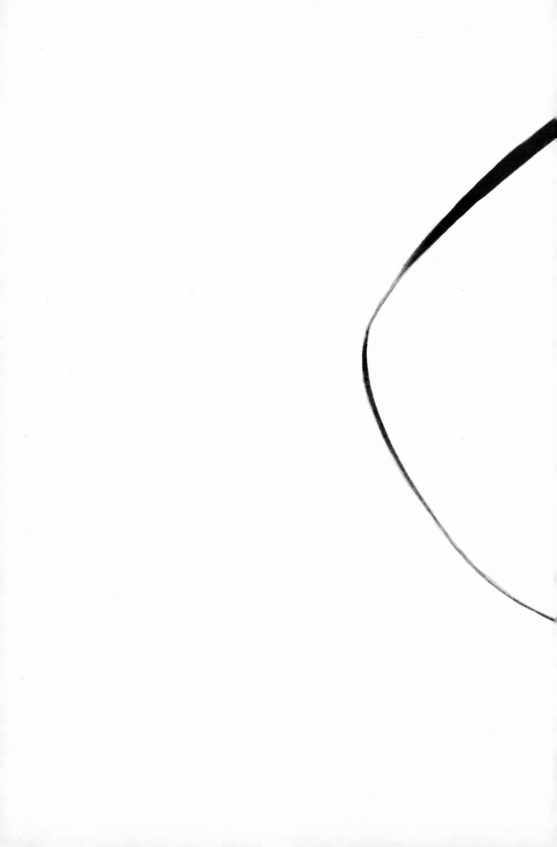

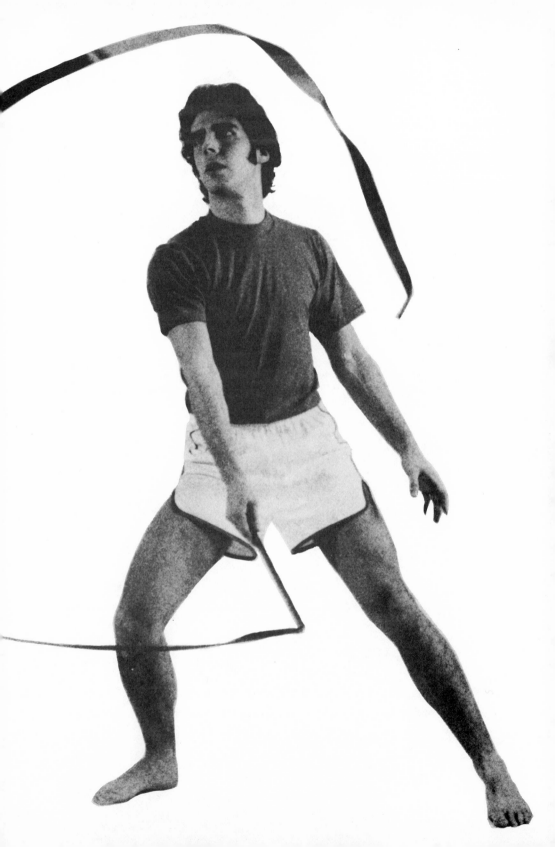

THREE

WAND EXERCISES FOR WEIGHT REDUCTION

A few years ago, a group of young Swedish women, the Sofia Girls, organized by a brilliant Swedish teacher of physical education, Maja Carlquist, presented a program of such beauty and delight that it had a profound influence on modern gymnastics. All who saw the Sofia Girls in action were eager to try the program.

Inspired by the Sofia Girls, the Royal Swedish Wand Exercises were designed not only to help trim away excess fat and to firm up sagging tissues, but to have very real muscle-toning and strengthening benefits for both sexes and all ages.

The technique is that of the Sofia Girls: one of muscular relaxation and a rhythmical execution of free-spirited calisthenics without tension. Its philosophy is the belief that physical development and fitness are as good for the mind as for the body.

Each wand exercise has its own image. Keep the image of each routine clear in your mind as you give full sway to your imagination. Visualize in technicolor the image of the routine.

The imagination is each person's bright flame, frequently snuffed out as we leave childhood to face the often grim realities and responsibilities of adulthood. Imagination is a muscle, too! It is the muscle of creativity, invention; it leads us from the walls of city life to the world of trees, mountains, seas or birds that fly like the wind.

Don't toss that precious muscle into the far recesses of your mind to gather dust. Use it, or it will, as will any muscle for lack of use, wither. Never feel guilty about your brief escape from the day's

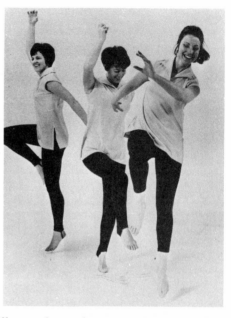

Bouncing in rhythm, a trio of Swedish officeworkers relieve tensions at group meetings where they follow the relaxing exercises developed by Swedish gymnasts.

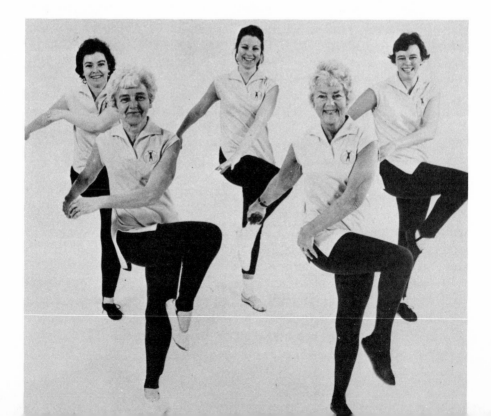

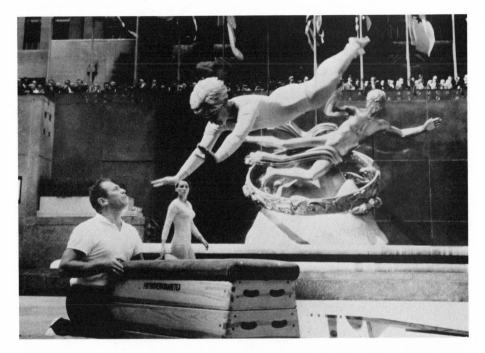

Flying dive is beautifully executed by Anita Jacobsson of the Sofia Girls during a 1967 performance of the group at Rockefeller Plaza in New York. Sofia Girls are world famous, but all began without any special aptitude for gymnastics.

Housewives young and not-so-young show the perfect control and joyous freedom that is the result of months of group training in one of the calesthenics groups.

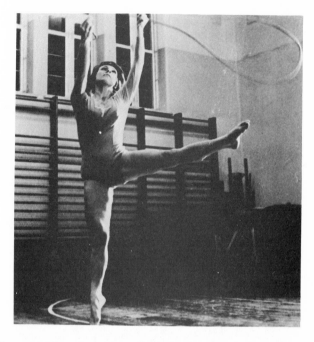

Wand exercise in action illustrated by one of Sweden's famous Sofia Girls. The purpose of the Sofia Girls' exercise is to improve physical fitness through muscular relaxation.

Balancing act performed by the Sofia Girls can be duplicated by anybody—but the physical fitness that makes it possible to hold this pose comfortably for extended periods is the result of persistent training, a fitness that brings your whole body beautifully under control.

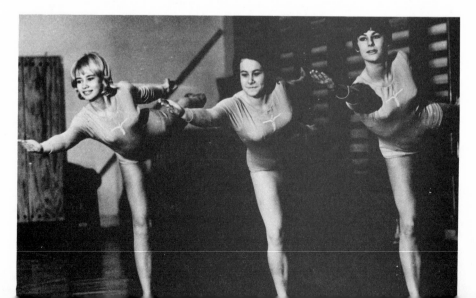

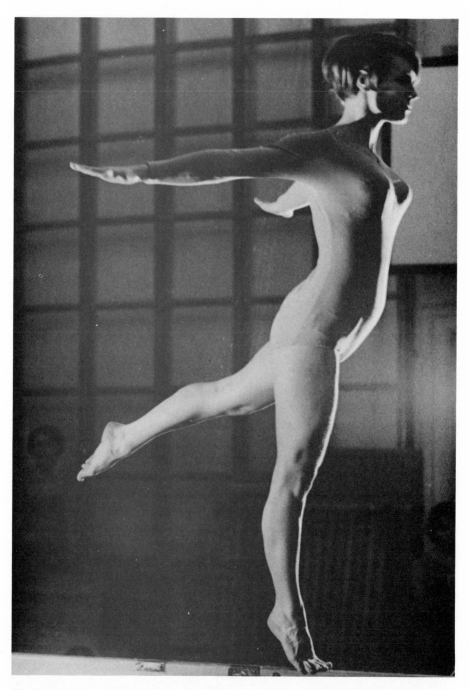

Rhythmical execution of exercises is the goal of Sweden's celebrated gymnastic teams. The philosophy behind the exercises is that physical development is as important to the mind as it is to the body.

pressures. Your dreaming can restore hope and rephrase your entire attitude, toward yourself, your work, and your world.

• Start the turning of your imaginative wheels as you swirl the wand with fluid movements to portray the image of the exercise.
• Perform your wand exercises to music! The emotional response to music is greater and more immediate than are any other responses of the senses.
• Use recordings or radio broadcasts of music that exhilarate you and make you want to move or to dance. Waltzes, polkas, tangos, folk songs, the scores of musical comedies, symphonies. Jazz or the classics. It doesn't matter what kind of music, so long as it gives you a sense of hope, pure pleasure, and not defeat or sadness.
• Progress smoothly and rhythmically from one exercise to another.
• Change the rhythm of your movements as the musical tempo changes.
• Use the scale of your emotions just as you use the range of your muscles. Let your emotions go from the gay and lively mood of the polka, to the softly romantic mood of the waltz, then to the moods of the ocean, fierce and strong!
• Repeat, several times and separately, the leg and torso movements and the wand patterns of each exercise.

Make these exercises the backbone, the mainstay of your personal physical fitness program. Once mastered, they will take only minutes from your day, wonderful, joyous minutes on which to build successful 24-hour blocks of work, play, and sleep.

For exercises that deal with specific needs and problems, use as your reference guide the chapters that follow. There are described comprehensive sets of exercises with specific purposes: the Royal Swedish way to remove spot bulges, preseason exercises for sportsmen, on-the-spot exercises devised for Swedish office workers and those in sedentary jobs, exercises to do as a group, a family, a twosome, tone-up routines for housewives, limber-up programs for older people. Work with whichever of these will solve the problem of the moment, then go back to your daily routine with the wand exercises. These will maintain the trim, limber you you've worked to achieve.

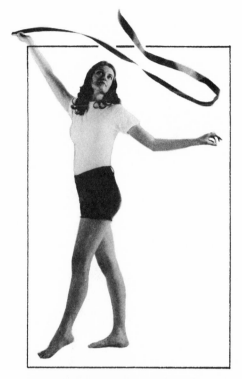

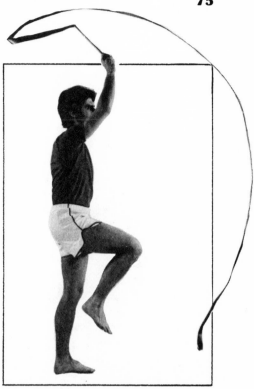

THE PRINCESS WALTZ

Music: Waltz
Wand Patterns: Ripples and Figure Eights

Rhythm
1. ONE Rt. Ft. forward; two Lt. Ft. forward to the left; three Rt. Ft. close to the left, and swirl wand ribbons to the right as you sway right.
   Change weight to Lt. Ft.
ONE Lt. Ft. forward; two Rt. Ft. forward to the right; three Lt. Ft. close to the right and swing left arm to the left as you sway left. Continually alternate wand-ribbon patterns.
   Change weight to Rt. Ft.
Continue by repeating waltz steps for one minute. (Waltz turn: Vary waltz step by pivoting on the ball of the foot that takes the step on the accented count "ONE.")

MARCH OF THE TROLLS

Music: March, Polka, or Cha-Cha
Wand Patterns: Horizontal Zigs and Vertical Zags

1. March in place, stepping high and lively, keeping in time to the music. Lift knees as high as you can, pointing toes downward, to stretch and slim calves, limber ankle joints, and strengthen thighs. Keep leg that carries body weight straightened and heels flat on the floor. Use full arm movements to create Horizontal Zigs and Vertical Zags as you alternate arms, thirty seconds with each arm. Walk forward four steps. Walk backward four steps. March around room, gradually increasing pace so that you are almost running. Gradually decrease pace until you are marching in place. As you exercise, alternate arms, thirty seconds with each arm.

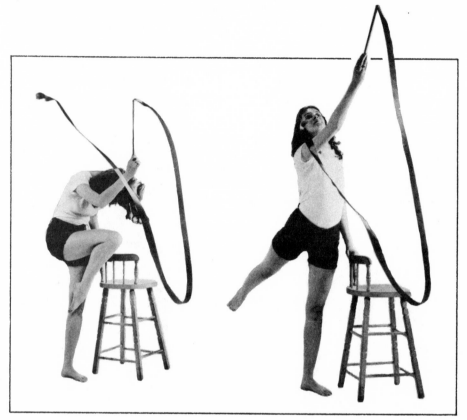

VAGEN
OCEAN WAVES

Music: Of your choice.
Wand Pattern: Ocean Waves

1. Support self with hand on a window ledge or sturdy chair. Place weight on left leg, arch body forward, chin down, as you lift your right knee up toward your chin, toe pointed. Wand in right hand. Each time the knee comes forward, the arm swings back. Swirl wand back and around.

2. Thrust leg back as you straighten your back and lift chest and chin. Swirl wand forward into crest of Ocean Wave pattern. Repeat, lifting the right knee, arching body forward. Swirl wand back, and continue pattern of Ocean Waves. Repeat sequence for 30 seconds; then perform sequence with left leg for 30 seconds. Use alternate arm when you perform exercise with left leg.

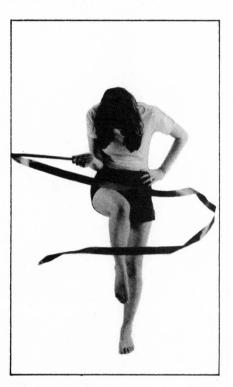

CANCAN JOG

Music: Gaiete Parisienne or other
brisk, lively melody
Wand Patterns: Small and large
Circles, Spirals, and the Wand Whip

1. Jog in place to Cancan tempo:
One - two - three - four, kick, kick.
Then, start with small Circles to the
sides and gradually increase size of
Circle patterns, then blend into
Spirals. Kick as high as you can with
each leg after each one-two-three-
four count. Use kicks as accent for
"cracking the Wand Whip."

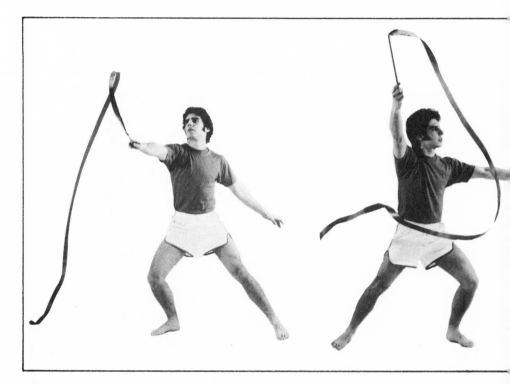

THE RAINBOW

Music: Of your choice.
Wand Patterns: Horizontal Arcs and
Figure Eights

1. Bend right knee as you lean
forward over right thigh. Keep back
straight and chest high as you lift
wand up high and forward. Swirl
wand ribbons in large Figure Eight
spirals.

2. Simultaneously straighten right
knee and lift right heel to

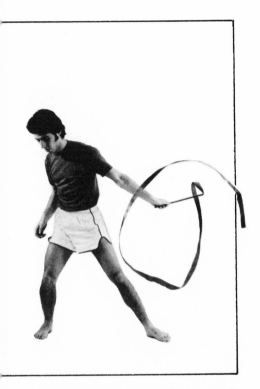

3. Pivot on right toe and sway to the left. Repeat, leaning on left leg. Alternately blend Horizontal Arcs with rainbow arcs of Figure Eight in a smooth, rhythmic flow. Change tempo from fast to slow, following musical tempo. Use a greater stretch during brisk musical passages.

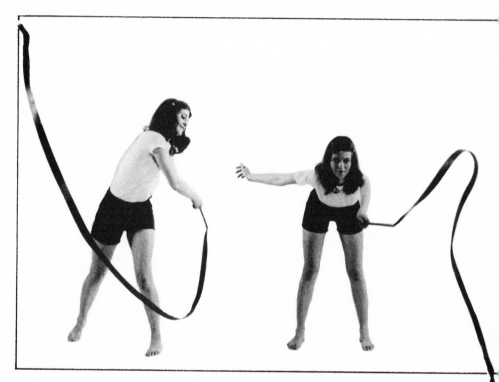

FLOD
THE RIVER

2. Turn front, bend forward and swirl wand forward in a giant arc.

Music: Of your choice.
Wand Patterns: Spirals, Arcs, Ripples

1. Stand with feet 12 inches apart. Without moving legs or hips, twist to the left from the waist up. Swirl wand ribbons in spiral pattern to the left, then twist to the right, spirals to the right.

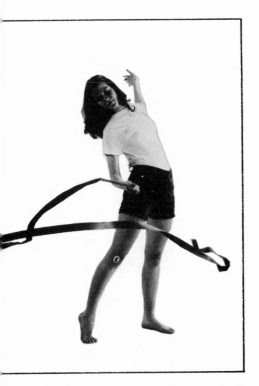

*3. Bend back; then whip wand rib-
bons back; then straighten, and blend
arc into ripple pattern. Repeat routine from left twist for one minute.
Continually blend one wand pattern
into the next.*

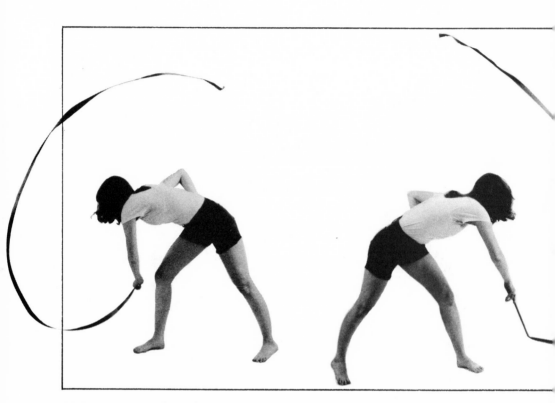

MOUNTAIN SPRINGS

Music: Selection from Musical Comedy, Waltz, or Tango.
Wand Patterns: Figure Eights, Wide Ripples, Arcs and Circles, and Ocean Waves

1. Right foot steps right. As you sway deeply to the right, swirl wand into one Figure Eight, left foot close to right foot. Right foot steps right. Blend Figure Eight into two wide ripples as

2. Left foot steps left. Sway deeply to the left, right foot close to left foot, left foot steps left, then blend into wide arc forward as

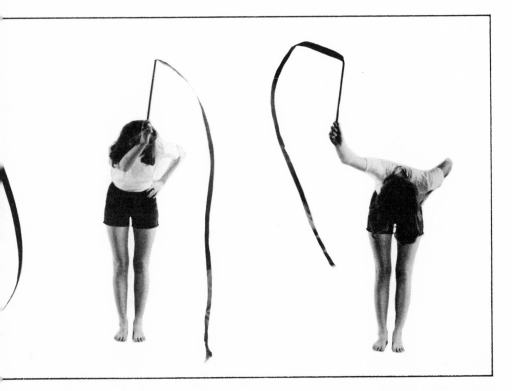

3. Right foot steps forward. Bend forward, back straight, left foot close forward to right foot. Right foot steps forward. Make two large Circles.

4. Left foot steps backward. Bend back, right foot close backward to left foot. Left foot steps backward. Repeat routine from 1 through 4.

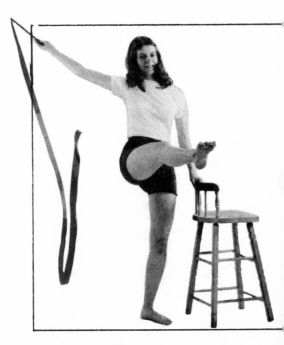

FISK MASEN
THE SEAGULL

Music: Selection from Musical Comedy, Folk Ballad, Waltz, or Opera Wand Patterns: Circles, Ocean Waves, Figure Eights, Ripples, and Spirals

1. Stand with both feet turned out, Chaplin-fashion. Slide heel of right foot alongside left foot so right foot is just in front of left, in the ballet "fifth position." Hold onto a sturdy chair for support. The following sequence should be done as one continual motion. Back straight, head up, lift leg to the front as high as you can as you circle wand ribbon's over head. Increase size of Circles, and lower leg to ballet fifth position; then gradually blend Circles into Ocean Waves, while you lift leg to the side.

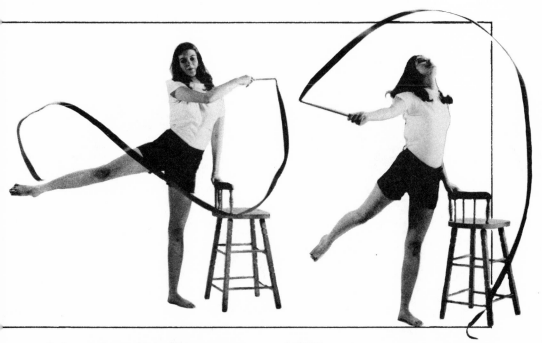

2. Lower leg to ballet fifth position as you blend Ocean Waves into horizontal Figure Eights. Lift leg to the back and up, making Ripples; lower leg to ballet fifth position. Without pausing, lift leg to the side and back to ballet fifth position while you make horizontal Spirals to the front, then giant horizontal Figure Eights, then Ripples; lift arms up and swirl wand into Circles above head. Rest, and turn and repeat whole sequence with alternate leg and arm.

NOTE:
Gradually try to increase height of kick, keeping knee straightened. For fun, improvise the wand swirls, using the ribbons to suggest the flight of the sea gull.

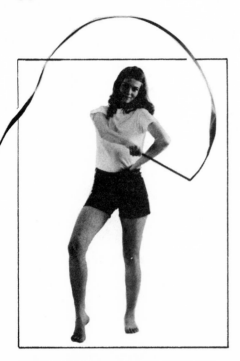
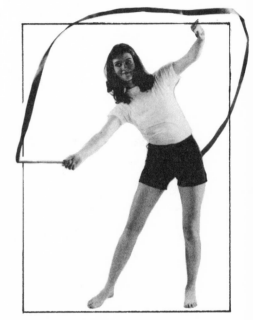

THE STOCKHOLM POLKA

Music: Polka, Cha-Cha or Schottische
Wand Patterns: Figure Eights, Circles, Ripples, and Horizontal Zags

1. *Weight on left foot, swirl wand into four figure eight patterns, as you tap floor with right heel; tap floor with right toe. Without pausing between patterns, step forward on right foot; swirl wand into circles; close left foot to right foot, then step forward on right foot. Ripple wand from side to side four times. Tap floor with left heel; and tap floor with left toe. Step forward with left foot; blend ripple patterns into two horizontal zags as you close right foot to left foot, step forward with left foot. Improvise wand patterns, changing combinations.*
NOTE:
Bend forward with first forward step, bend to the right with second forward step and to the left with the next forward step, alternating bending with each step forward.

VATTEVFALL
THE WATERFALL

Music: Musical-Comedy Selection, Tango, or Folk Tune.
Wand Patterns: Arcs, Ripples, and Circles

1. *Stand with legs wide apart, arms extended at sides, shoulder level. Wand in right hand. Lead with wrist as you swing right arm above head to the left, arching upper torso. Lift with the upswing of the arm. Bend left knee slightly; keep right leg straightened. Bounce gently to the left three times. Blend into Ripple patterns right and left across your body at the waist. Slowly straighten left knee as you return to upright position, swinging wand in an Arc back over your head, leading with the inner wrist as you return to upright position. Blend Arc into Circles, and continue into arc pattern as you repeat sequence. Repeat exercise, bending to right and swinging left arm above head and to the right. Continue arching body to each side for one minute.*

PART III
EXERCISES TO MEET
SPECIAL NEEDS

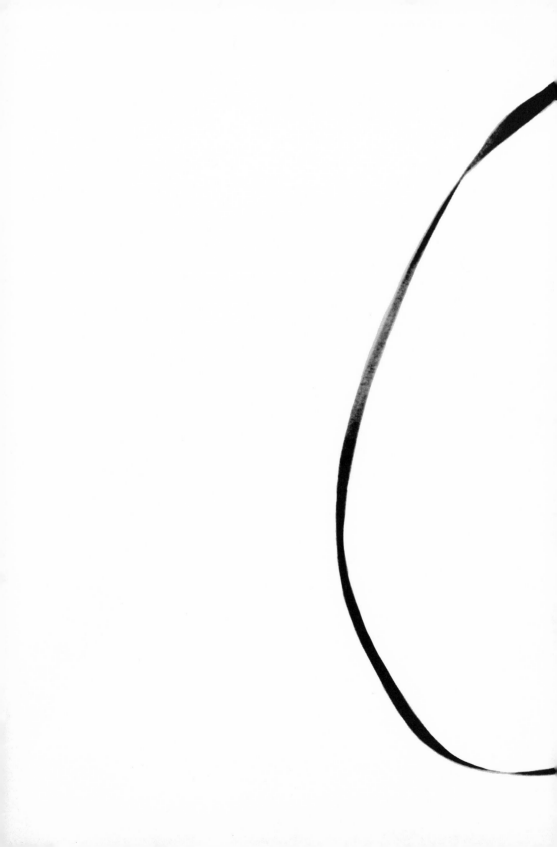

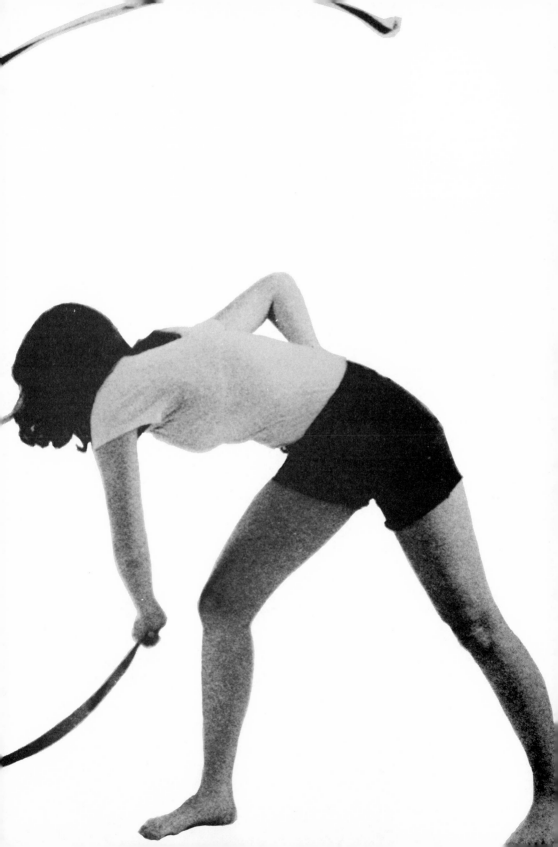

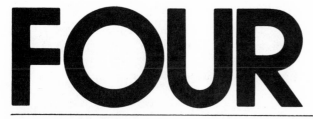

EXERCISES
FOR SPOT CONTROL

You are not alone when you see in a mirror portions of your body you wish were smaller, firmer, or fuller. Almost everyone does. This may be only your own harsh estimate of yourself, but frequently there are areas that should and can be improved.

Spot control exercises provide the means of effecting such correctives through (a) muscular toning and strengthening and (b) dissolving cellulite deposits.

Cellulite deposits are those rippling wads of fatty tissue that plague both men and women. This needless fat is pocketed mostly along the inner thighs, the knees, abdomen, buttocks, upper arms and legs. It is not inevitable with age. Cellulite is primarily the result of improper diet and little or no exercise.

Most of the exercises below are suggested for a limited daily corrective session. Once the problems are corrected, a daily routine of wand exercises will keep you lithe and slim.

Bear in mind, constantly, that the good from these exercises should not be derived at the expense of your physical well-being or through complete exhaustion. If instructions call for repeating an exercise six times and you're tired at four, call a halt. Stay with four until you can easily bring it up to five and then six.

The change in you won't happen all at once. There will be periods of discouragement, even of seeming retrogression. Stick with your regimen, enjoy the graceful, gradual strengthening, firming, correcting that these exercises will bring you. There will come a magic moment when you realize that those unwanted inches are gone, that what was flabby has become firm, that you've made very definite, discernible progress toward becoming the you you want to be.

Few discoveries you'll ever make will prove that gratifying!

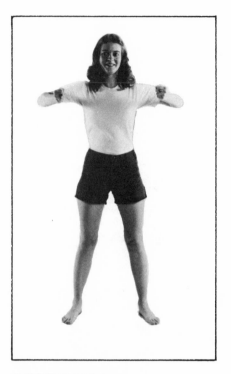

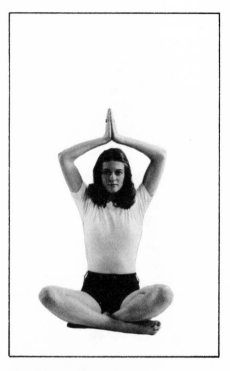

SPOT CONTROL
for Shoulders

GOALS:
To trim down dowager's hump at the back of neck and shoulders.

START:
Stand with legs shoulders' width apart. Arms are bent and raised shoulder level; fists clenched.
1. Inhale as you lift elbows just above shoulder level. Exhale as you thrust shoulders back as hard as you can. Hold this position for five counts. Then inhale, slowly bringing elbows forward to return to starting position. Repeat entire sequence ten times.

SPOT CONTROL
for Pectoral Muscles

GOALS:
To firm and strengthen pectoral muscles.

START:
This exercise may be done lying on your back anywhere, sitting or standing.
1. Whether lying on back, sitting or standing, contract abdomen and lift hands above your head. Flex elbows slightly and touch fingertips of both right and left hands to each other, steeple fashion. Inhale, and press fingertips against each other as firmly as you can, with almost a pushing motion. Exhale as you release fingertip pressure. Repeat 12 times as often during the day as you can.

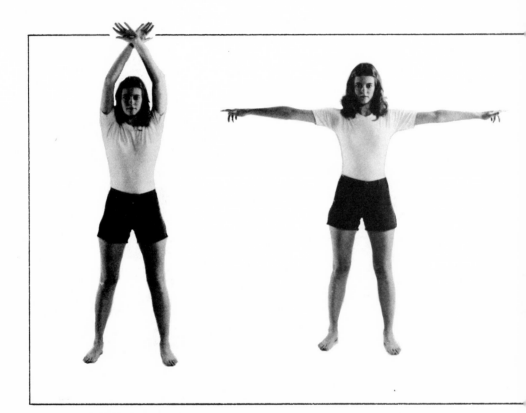

SPOT CONTROL for Arms

GOALS:
To tighten sag in arms and armpits, train arm and shoulder muscles; improve nutrition of articular cartilage.

START:
Stand, arms relaxed at sides.
NOTE:
This exercise should be performed with contracted inner-arm muscles; relax at conclusion of sequence.
1. Lift arms, and cross wrists above head, elbows rounded.

2. Uncross wrists, and swing arms down to shoulder level; bounce extended arms as far back as you can without strain, three times. Then

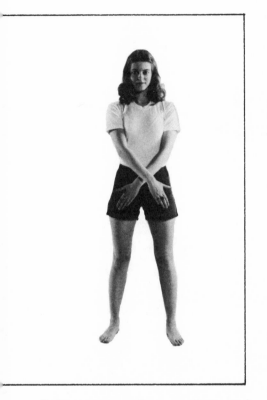

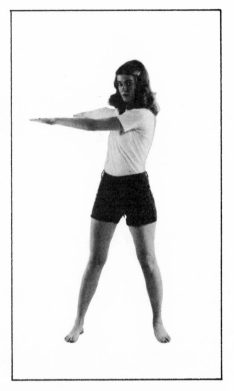

3. Continue to swing arms down and cross wrists in front of you and swing arms up again to 1 position. Relax tension in arms as you return to Starting Position, and rest for six counts. Repeat complete exercise five times.

SPOT CONTROL
for Waist

GOALS:
To firm waistline and hips.

START:
Stand, legs wide apart, arms relaxed at sides.
1. Bend right knee slightly, with weight on right leg. Twist at the waist to the right as you swing both arms to the right, just above shoulder level.
2. Swing arms down, from right, across body, to the left; simultaneously, twist body from waist to left, straightening the right knee and bending the left as you turn. As both arms come up the left side, shift body weight to the left knee. Repeat half-circle pendulum arm-swing from one side to the other, twisting from right to left and back, ten times.

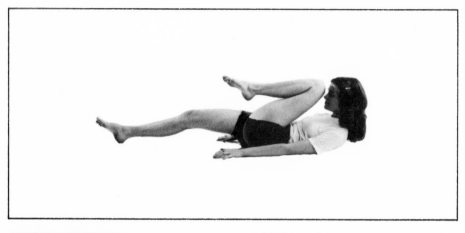

SPOT CONTROL
for Abdomen

GOALS:
To trim hips, strengthen abdominal muscles and back.

START:
Lie on back on floor.
1. Alternately raise right and left leg as you bring upper torso forward to meet knee with the forehead. Feel the contraction of your abdominal muscles. Continue for 15 seconds. Rest for 30 seconds after each fifteen-second stint. Repeat until slightly tired.

LATER, after abdominal muscles have strengthened:
1. Raise both legs and your arms, balancing yourself. Then, vertebra by vertebra, slowly lower your body until you press lower back against floor.

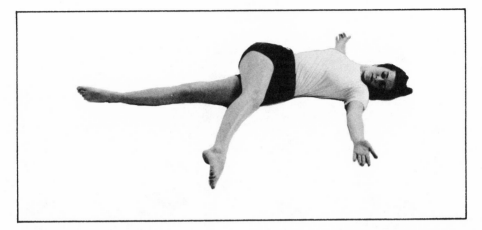

SPOT CONTROL
for Hips and Waist

GOALS:
To trim and tone hips and waistline.

START:
Lie with your lower back pressed against the floor. Arms are outstretched on the ground on either side, at shoulder level, palms up. Legs are fourteen inches apart.

1. Extend right leg straight up and over, across left leg, pointing toe to the left. Keep palms up, arms extended, shoulders flattened against the floor. Return right leg across left leg to starting position, keeping knee straight, then repeat exercise with left leg. Return to starting position. Repeat entire exercise eight times.

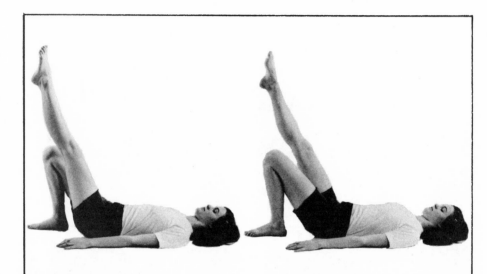

SPOT CONTROL
for Buttocks and Hips

GOALS:
To trim buttocks and hips.

START:
Lie on back, arms relaxed at sides, palms down.
1. Bend right knee and slide foot along floor until right heel is on the floor, close to buttocks.

2. Lift left leg, knee straightened, and point toe toward ceiling. Pull leg up as high as you comfortably can. Bounce leg up three times to reach a high-kick position. Then slowly relax pull, and lower left leg slowly. Keep knee straight until your heel has reached the floor. Straighten bent right knee, and bring up left knee as in sequence 1. Repeat 2, lifting and lowering right leg. Straighten bent left knee, and return to starting position. Repeat entire exercise five times.

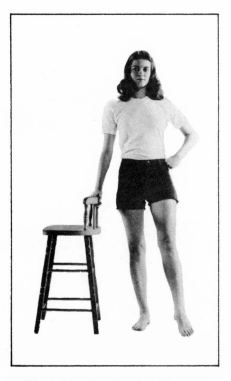

SPOT CONTROL for Knees

GOALS:
To reduce fatty knee bulge, trim hips.

START:
Stand beside a chair, low mantel, towel bar, dresser or other heavy furniture, with right hand on this support, left arm extended to the side at shoulder level.
1. Place weight on right leg. Lift left leg about four inches from the floor and draw ten circles with your toe pointed toward the ground. Turn around; place weight on left leg, and hold with your left hand. Draw ten circles with your right toe. Repeat complete exercise ten times.

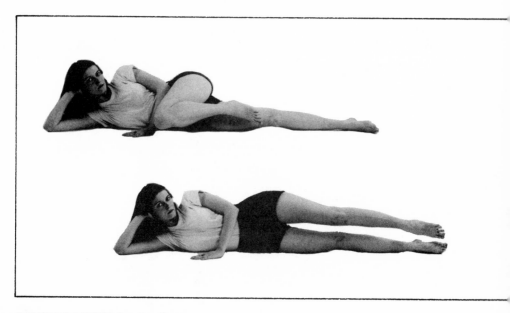

SPOT CONTROL for Legs

2. Straighten leg.

GOALS:
To firm waist, trim hips, buttocks, thighs, and legs. An excellent, all-over trim-down routine.

START:
Lie on floor, on your right side. Rest on right arm, bent at the elbow. Steady yourself with the palm of your left hand in front of you on the floor. 1. Lift left leg, bend knee, and bring knee close to body.

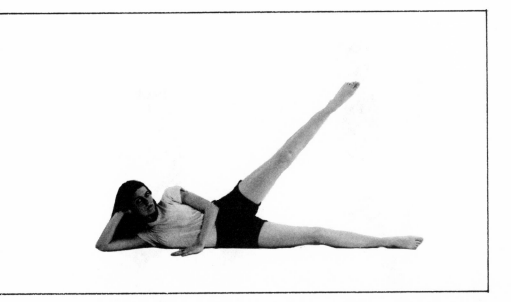

3. Lift it as high as you can, pointing toe toward ceiling. Lower leg, and resume bent-knee position in 1, and return to starting position, lowering bent knee. Raise leg again; this time, as high as you can and back from hips a little. Point toe and draw six eight-inch circles forward and six circles backward. Return leg to starting position. Repeat five times. Turn on left side, and repeat entire sequence with right leg. Lie on your back, arms extended above head and rest.

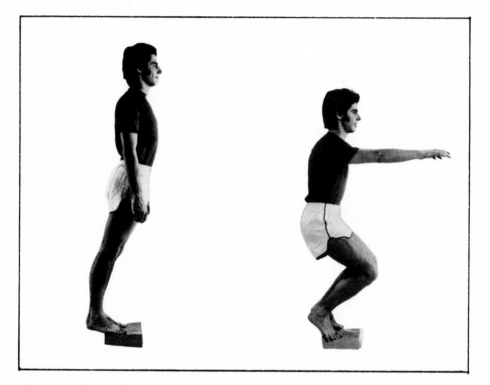

SPOT CONTROL
for Legs and Ankles

GOALS:
To firm legs and ankles.

START:
Stand with balls of feet, each on the edge of a thick book. Select two books of approximately the same thickness. Hold on to a chair back or the sides of a doorway. Or you may stand with balls of feet on the edge of a bottom step; face the staircase.

1. Holding on to chair, doorway or banisters for safety, rise on your toes and hold position for a count of two. Lower your heels to just below book or stair level. Repeat ten times.

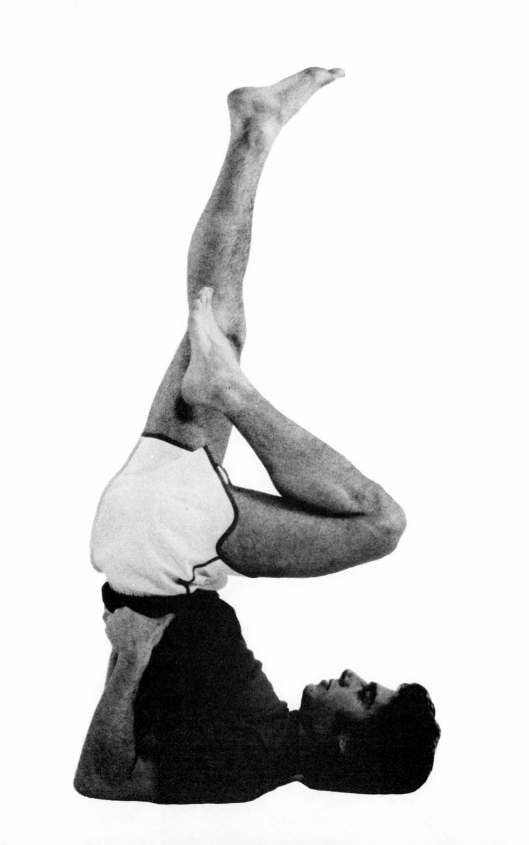

FIVE

EXERCISES FOR SPORTSMEN

Effective performance of all active sports depends heavily on the muscles to provide the Big Four: strength, endurance, agility, and mobility.

This chapter comprises a conditioning and strengthening program for all those who participate in active sports. The exercises are more advanced than those presented previously because the needs of the athlete's body to respond quickly and efficiently to demands are considerably greater.

The key word here is balance. Do not sacrifice one part of the body to overdevelop another.

Your sports program is constructed so that the four major aspects of good athletic performance are covered. To achieve necessary mobility—the ability to perform your chosen sport fluidly, without strain—use the limbering exercises in Chapter II: Swedish Limber-Up Exercises.

To gain greater agility and quickness, select the exercises you require to develop the muscle groups needed for your sport. In many sports speed is not as important as quickness. A person who has sheer speed may not be able to defeat an opponent on a tennis or handball court, where the play area is limited, if his opponent can start or stop fast enough and possesses swift lateral range.

He might be able to defeat that opponent handily in a 100-yard dash, but for the 27- or 36-yard width of a tennis court, he might be more than equally matched. It depends on the sport. In a game like soccer or rugby, pure speed would be much more important because the size of the playing area is large.

Strength and power are substantial attributes, but they shouldn't be developed at the expense of endurance and mobility. Nor is power a direct function of strength. Power is the efficient application of force and often requires experience and intelligence, rather than simple muscle capacity. Weight lifting and isometrics can be a valuable asset to sports conditioning. This is especially true in contact sports, where strength and muscle play an important role. But it is not necessary to lift weights for all sports, just as it is unnecessary to strive for brute strength in all sports.

If an athlete specializes in one activity, such as bowling or tennis or skiing, frequently just repeating the movements the sport requires may give him all the power he needs. Some athletes, such as track men, swimmers, and golfers, may actually avoid weight training because they believe that weight lifting hinders the smoothness of their stride or stroke.

Endurance, the body's capacity to delay muscle fatigue, is one of the most vital but overlooked aspects of athletic performance. There are countless examples of two evenly matched contestants playing to a virtual stand-off, the winner being the one who lasts longer.

The ability to perform efficiently over a long period is a factor in every conceivable sport. There are no shortcuts to good conditioning. The only way an athlete can keep in shape is by exercising regularly and consistently. The type and intensity of exercise depend on the athlete's chosen sport and the degree of his involvement in it.

A weekend touch-football participant doesn't have to train as does a member of an Olympic ice-skating team. A sport such as water-skiing doesn't require the stamina needed to play handball.

There are many ways for an athlete to condition himself. The most effective is running. And the easiest form of running, but one never to be scoffed at by the sportsman, is . . .

JOGGING

On your first day of training—you should begin a training schedule at least three or four weeks prior to actual sports participation—rise early. Put on loose clothing and rubber-soled canvas shoes, and jog slowly around your garden or up and down the street. It doesn't matter if you hardly lift your legs as long as only one foot is on the ground at a time.

After you have jogged (however heavily, however slowly) up and down the block once, call it a day. Return home, and "warm down" with light limbering exercises. This will keep the muscles from cramping.

Repeat the slow jog on the second day. The third day you will be able to jog twice around the garden or twice up and down the street —even around the block. Each day you can add more distance and more speed, with less and less effort. Don't look now, but you're learning to breathe again!

If you are past the slow-jog stage, try varying your training schedule. Some days run steadily for a long period or over half an hour. On alternate days, try the *fartlek* routine devised by Swedish coaches for their world-class runners. *Fartlek* means speed-play, which is precisely what you do. Start with a comfortable jog for a quarter of a mile. Then increase your speed to a steady stride for 50 yards or approximately 12 seconds.

Then, for 25 yards, stride as fast as you can without straining. After you have reached the 25-yard mark, slow down to a sedate jog. Jog slowly until you have recovered your breath; then pick up your normal jogging pace, and repeat the entire *fartlek* procedure. This "playing" at different speeds has been found to accustom an athlete to the periodic bursts of speed necessary in many sports that demand a quick-start and quick-stop technique.

Wind sprints are short-distance running spurts, or dashes. Short sprints, from 20 to 70 yards, alternated with brief rest periods, are outstanding conditioners. Take repeated wind sprints for 50 yards.

Walk one minute between sprints. Do not stop moving. Start with two sprints, and work up to ten. You will gradually need less rest time between sprints as your lungs become stronger. The less rest and the shorter the rest periods, the faster your lungs will strengthen.

After a few weeks, try jogging between sprints. Then perform a few limbering exercises for a warm-down.

ARRANGING YOUR SPORTS EXERCISE PROGRAM

- Precede every exercise program with limbering (or warm-up) exercises. A good warm-up will lessen fatigue and eliminate debilitating muscle cramps and pulls that cause needless accidents.
- Inspect the Sport and Body-Movement Index on page 123.Note the sport of your choice; then follow the column on the left to learn which parts of the body are involved. Then look up the exercises to make certain they cover a muscle group used in your sport. Include the exercises in your program, but
- Be selective. You do not have to perform every listed exercise each day.
- Stretching exercises should be performed daily. Developing or strengthening exercises may be done on alternating days.
- Perform this RELAXATION after each exercise:
  Stand limply. Lean against the wall with your right hand. Raise the left leg just off the floor. Keep your knee released and free as you wiggle the foot loosely from the ankle. Turn, and repeat with the right leg. Then stand in a broad stride, and let the upper torso hang forward, bent at the waist. Let both arms hang limply. Relax, rag-doll fashion, with shoulders, arms, wrists, and hands dangling. Loll your neck and head forward and down. Swing from side to side in lazy-pendulum fashion for one minute.
- Perform even your sports exercises rhythmically, to music, the Swedish way. Even a topnotch football player has the grace of a ballet dancer and a pantherlike coordination.
- Keep a record of your exercise routine each day by listing the exercises and the number of times you performed them.

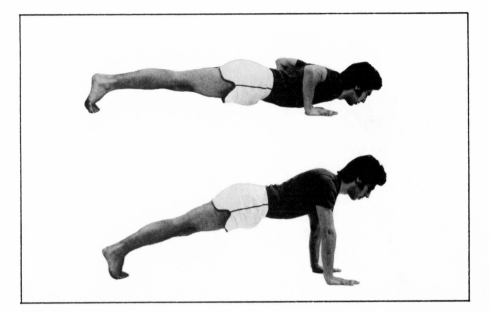

PUSH-UPS

GOALS:
To strengthen arms and shoulders and promote greater lung capacity. Avoid, if you are an out-of-training middle-ager, or if you suffer from hypertension.

START:
Lie on the floor, face down. Place palms on the floor, just under the shoulders, as in standard push-ups. 1. Holding the body rigid and the back perfectly straight, keep knees on the floor as you push up until the arms are fully extended.

2. Bend your elbows as your slowly lower the upper torso until chest touches the floor. Repeat twice. Work up gradually, each day, until you do at least ten.

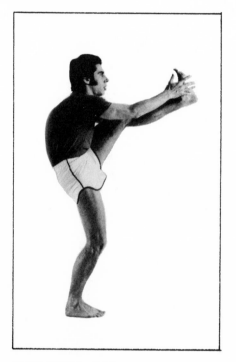

HIGH LEG KICK

GOALS:
To stretch hamstrings. Athletes and coaches consider this exercise one of the best and safest hamstring stretchers. This is designed for soccer, skiing, sports that require a lot of running; also for football and basketball.

START:
Stand with legs shoulders' width apart. Hands on hips.
1. Kick up as high as you can, pointing toes, and reach forward with extended arms to touch your toes at the highest point of the kick. Try to keep your head erect. Repeat twice with the right leg, then alternate legs. Get the greatest extension out of the kick for the greatest stretch.

STATIONARY RUN AND TURN

GOALS:
To create endurance and improve agility for basketball, tennis, handball.

START:
Stand arms bent at elbows, with forearms parallel to the floor. The object of this exercise is to run continually in place as rapidly as possible, raising knees high.
1. Start counting deliberately up to eight, turning on each second count: One-two — Turn while running, quarter turn to the left; Three-four — Turn while running, quarter turn back to the front; Five-six — Turn while running, quarter turn to the right; Seven-eight — Turn while running, quarter turn back to the front.
2. Continue running and repeat this sequence two more times. Without stopping, proceed to the next sequence, still running in place and still counting. One-two — On second count, without turning, run sideways to the right, four feet. Three-four — Without turning, run sideways back to center. Five-six — Without turning, run sideways left, four feet. Seven-eight — Without turning, run sideways back to center.

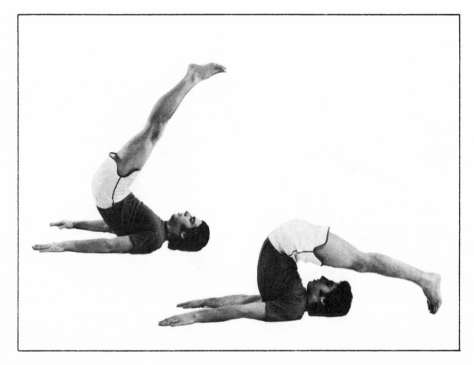

THE PLOW

GOALS:
Do this exercise once daily to gain trunk flexibility and to loosen the back. This is great for such sports as golf, tennis, skiing, and handball or paddleball, where reach and trunk flexibility are important.

START:
Lie on your back, arms on the floor at your sides.
1. Lift both legs, keeping them as straight as possible.

2. Bring legs up and over the head, so that your toes rest above your head on the floor. (When you do this exercise for the first time, you probably can't touch the floor; but it is important to keep the legs straight as you move them back as far as you can. Courage. You will grow more limber each day.) Hold this position, breathing very deeply, for 30 seconds. Stiffen knees, and bring your legs back over your head and down. Rest!

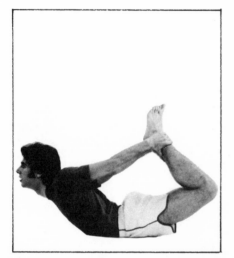

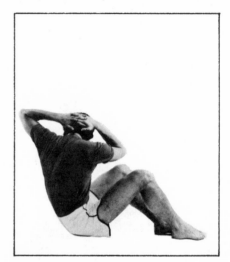

BACK ARCH AND ROLL

GOALS:
To loosen shoulders and thighs and strengthen the lower back. For golf, tennis, skiing.

START:
Lie on stomach. Bend knees so that lower legs are perpendicular to the floor.
IMPORTANT:
Breathe deeply and regularly to derive full benefit from this exercise.
1. Reach behind you and take hold of your right ankle with your right hand, left ankle with left hand. Arch back so that your chest and pelvis are off the floor, and rock back and forth six times. Relax. Release ankles. Rest for five counts and repeat.

SIT UP AND TWIST

GOALS:
To increase back and trunk suppleness. (You'll have even better results if this is done on a slantboard. This exercise is also an excellent stomach flattener.) This is good for skiing, tennis, golf.

START:
Lie on your back, hands behind your head, knees slightly bent. Anchor your feet under a heavy piece of furniture so you can't tip over while you're doing the exercise.
1. Sit up as you would normally, but when you reach the sitting position, twist the trunk rapidly to the left. Try to twist as fully to the side as possible. Lie back down, then repeat, this time turning vigorously to the right. Repeat this whole sequence 15 to 20 times.

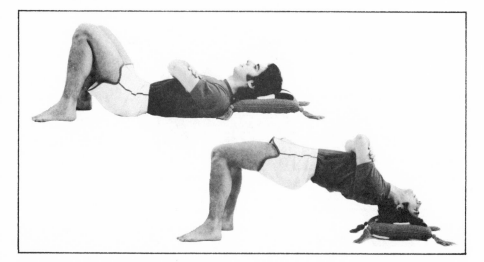

WRESTLER'S BRIDGE

GOALS:
To strengthen neck, firm thighs and abdomen, lower back. Good for contact sports, such as football and rugby.

START:
Lie on your back with a pillow behind your head. Fold your arms in front of your chest.
1. Bend your knees and position your feet flat on the floor, about 16 inches apart.

2. Arch your back and neck so that your body forms a bridge, supported by your feet at one end and the top of your head at the other. Hold this position while you count 104, 105, 106, 107. Relax. Lower your shoulders and back to the floor. Repeat this entire sequence three times.

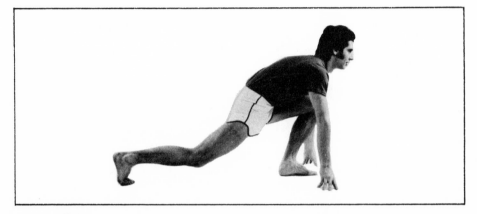

THE LEAN
AND THE SCISSORS

GOALS:
To stretch thigh and groin muscles. This exercise is outstanding as an agility drill. This is good for skiing, skating, baseball or softball, basketball, football.

START:
Stand with your feet together, arms at your sides.

1. Bring left leg forward, and bend left knee. Lean over, and place the tips of your fingers on the floor on each side of your left foot. Change leg positions quickly, retaining bent position of body: right leg forward, left leg back; right leg back, left leg forward. Continue until you start to tire.
NOTE:
Move arms as little as possible.

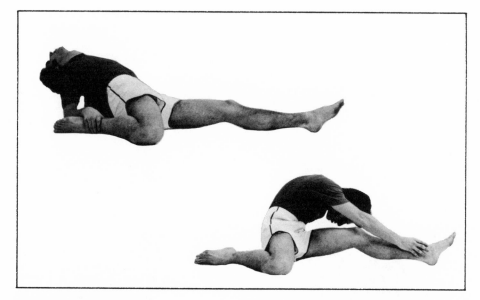

GROUND HURDLE

GOALS:
To stretch trunk. One of the most difficult but effective exercises, this is an all-purpose stretcher for trunk, hamstrings, thighs and calves. This is good for tennis, handball, swimming, basketball.

START:
Sit on floor with left leg extended straight in front of you. Bend right leg back so that the ankle is tucked in next to the buttocks.
1. Lean back as far as possible, feeling the stretch in the right thigh. Gently hold the right ankle with your right hand while doing so.

2. Lean forward, turning the trunk slightly. Try to touch your right hand to the toes of the extended left foot, bringing the head forward and down, as close to the left knee as possible. Bounce gently eight times. Alternate leg positions and repeat entire sequence.

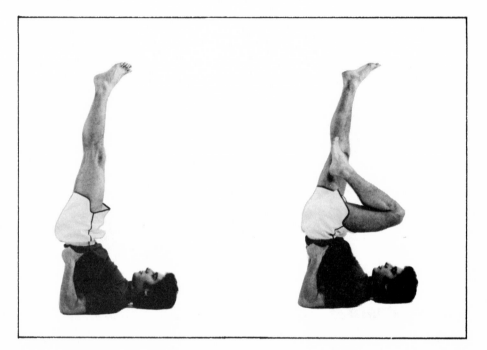

CYCLING - NO HANDS

GOALS:
To strengthen abdominal muscles and lower back. This is beneficial for those who play soccer, skate and ski cross-country.

START:
Lie on the floor on your back.
1. Lift legs so body is straight and vertical. Support upper back with arms. Elbows are resting on floor.

2. "Cycle" slowly forward twenty times, then back, twenty times. Gradually double the number of times of both forward and backward cycling.

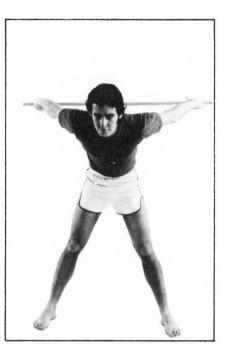

SHOULDER STRETCH

GOALS:
To loosen and limber muscles in chest, shoulders and arms. Good for golf, tennis, swimming, handball, paddleball.

START:
Stand with feet wide apart but firmly balanced. Hold a golf club or tennis racket horizontally behind you.
1. Bend over, keeping your head up, and raise your arms behind you, as high as possible. Bounce arms up toward your head five times. Relax and repeat three times.

SPORTS EXERCISE RECORD

EXER-CISE	Mon.	Tues.	Wed.	Thurs.	Fri.	Sat.	Sun.
1							
2							
3							
4							
5							
6							
7							
8							
9							
10							
11							
12							
13							
14							
15							

SPORT AND BODY-MOVEMENT INDEX

Stretch	Strengthen		Bicycling	Bowling	Canoeing	Diving	Golf	Handball	Skating	Skiing	Surfing	Swimming	Tennis	Water-skiing
	+	Hands & Arms	✓	✓	✓	✓	✓	✓		✓	✓	✓	✓	✓
	+	Shoulders	✓	✓	✓	✓	✓	✓		✓	✓	✓	✓	✓
	+	Chest				✓					✓	✓	✓	✓
0	+	Abdomen				✓	✓	✓	✓	✓	✓	✓	✓	✓
0	+	Upper Back	✓	✓	✓	✓	✓	✓	✓	✓	✓	✓	✓	
0	+	Lower Back	✓	✓		✓	✓	✓	✓	✓	✓	✓	✓	✓
	+	Gluteals (buttocks)	✓			✓	✓	✓	✓	✓	✓	✓	✓	✓
	+	Pelvis	✓			✓	✓	✓	✓	✓	✓	✓	✓	✓
0		Groin*		✓										
0	+	Thighs*	✓	✓		✓	✓	✓	✓	✓	✓	✓	✓	✓
0		Hamstrings*		✓	✓	✓			✓	✓	✓	✓	✓	✓
0	+	Calves	✓	✓		✓	✓	✓	✓	✓	✓	✓	✓	✓
0		Achilles Tendon*	✓			✓	✓		✓	✓	✓	✓	✓	✓
0	+	Ankles	✓	✓		✓	✓	✓	✓	✓	✓	✓	✓	✓
0	+	Arches		✓		✓		✓	✓	✓			✓	

* used in all running activities

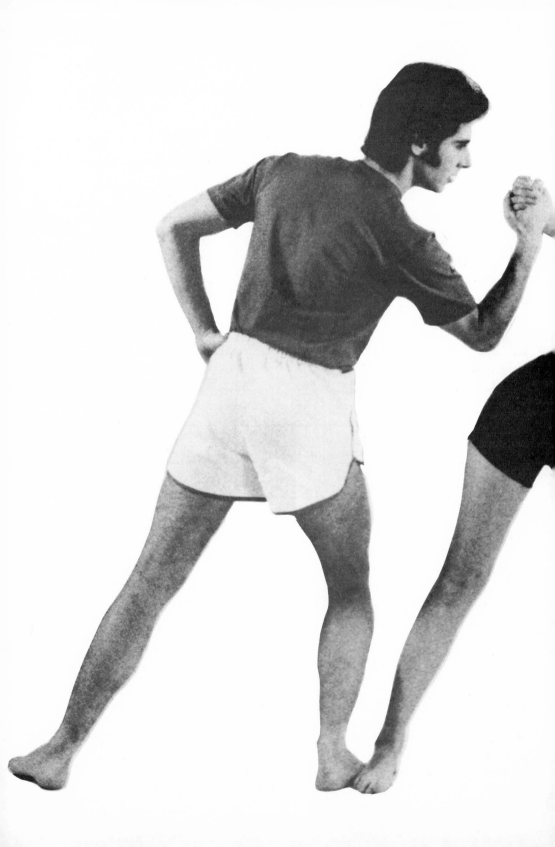

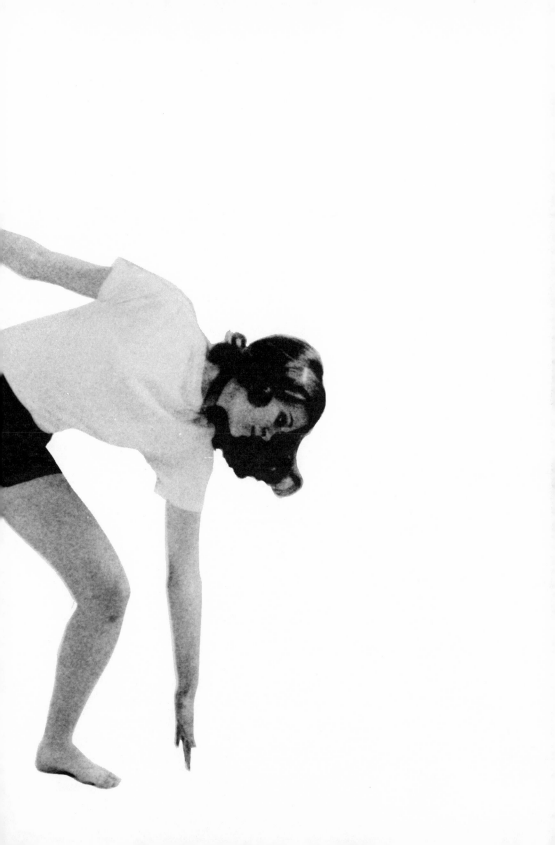

SIX

EXERCISES TO DO TOGETHER

The Royal Swedish Exercises are especially rewarding when a group works together. Here is a potpourri of exercises suggested by the beautiful Berit Brattnäs Stanton, Sports Attache for the Swedish Consulate General, who has done much to introduce us to the Royal Swedish Way of exercising.

There are special Exercises for Two, Pausgymnastik (office exercise breaks), Husmorgymnastiken (fitness for housewives); and the Medelalders och Aldre training program, an exercise regimen suggested by the noted Dr. Per-Olof Astrand that has become a way of life for thousands of Swedish people of middle age.

EXERCISES FOR TWO

These exercises may be performed by members of a family, friends, parents and children, husbands and wives. They might even be called Love Plays because their importance depends not on how one partner can surpass the other, but on how well each can respond to the other so they work as a unit—the key to people-living.

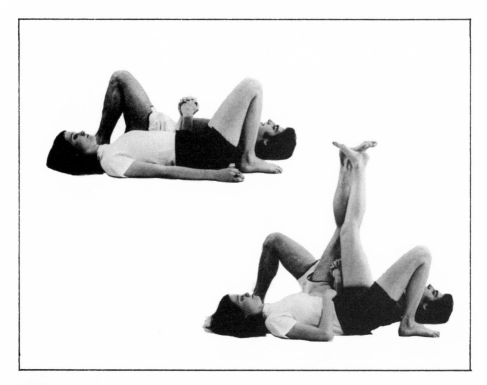

VIKING OARSMEN

GOALS:
Keeping the rhythms of rowing a boat with the leg lifts stretches and tightens abdomen.

START:
A and B (or groups of two) lie on the floor facing in opposite directions, adjacent lower arms entwined.
1. Bend the outer knee with the heel close to the buttocks, foot flat on the floor.

2. Simultaneously, A and B lift straightened inside leg as high as possible, and their ankles touch. Then each lowers leg to the floor and quickly lifts it again. Repeat rapidly 20 times, lifting leg, touching ankles, and lowering leg. Partners should keep in rhythmic pace. Turn about, and repeat exercise, using alternate legs.

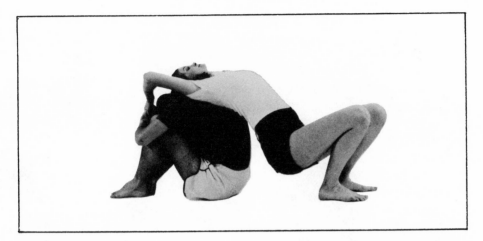

HIP ROLL

GOALS:
To trim hips, strengthen abdomen.

START:
A and B sit on floor, back to back. Both extend arms above head. A reaches back to clasp hands of B.

1. A bends forward, bringing arms, torso, and chest towards knees, pulling B up slightly from the seated position. A holds position for two counts, then lowers B slowly, returning to upright position and simultaneously lifting arms above head. B repeats sequence, bending forward as in 1 and 2. Each partner alternately bends for one minute. Be gentle!

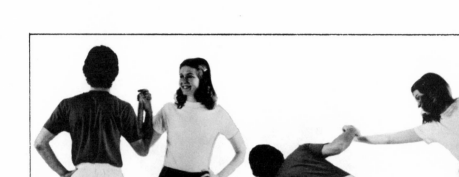

ROCKING

GOALS:
To trim waist fat and tighten thigh muscles.

START:
A and B stand side by side, facing in opposite directions, legs wide apart. Outer side of A's right foot touches outer side of B's right foot; A's right hand clasps B's right hand. Both partners extend the left arm to the side, shoulder level.

1. A bends to the side, supported by B, to touch floor, then straightens as
2. B bends to the side, supported by A, to touch the floor, then straightens.
NOTE:
Each partner uses a resistive support for the side bend of the other as he reaches to touch the floor.

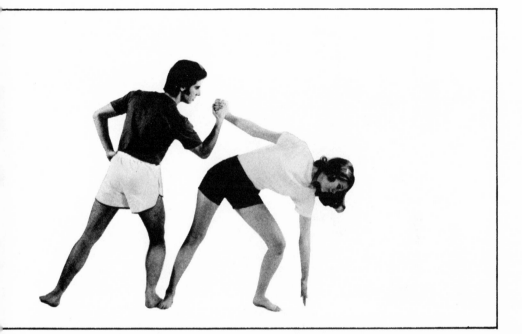

3. Partners alternately repeat side bend ten times. Then

4. Turn about: A and B turn so left feet touch and left hands are clasped. Now, going in opposite directions from 1 and 2 they alternately touch the floor, ten times.
TIME:
One minute.

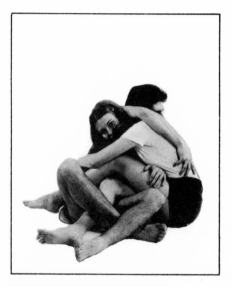

THE LOVERS' KNOT

GOALS:
To improve endurance and flexibility.

START:
A and B sit on floor, intertwine legs and arms in helter-skelter fashion, and clasp hands. The arms and legs of each partner are loosely intertwined with the others but each should be sure that no strain is involved.
1. Responding to the movement of the partner, both simultaneously rise from the floor, disentangling enough to attain a standing position, but still keeping the hands joined. With hands still clasped, melt into each other, turning and interlocking and descend slowly to the floor.
NOTE:
The possibilities of this exercise, visually and physically, are hilarious and wonderful! Two points must be kept in mind: hand contact must never be broken, and a responsiveness and a giving attitude must be maintained.

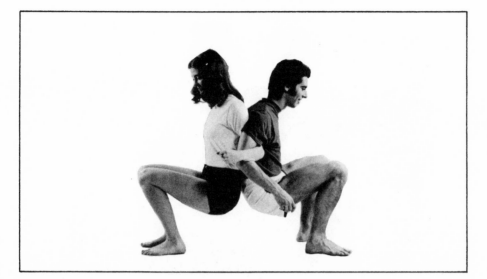

RISING OF TROLLS

GOALS:
Trim thighs and strengthen leg muscles.

START:
A and B sit on the floor, back to back, knees bent, feet flat on the floor with heels just under thighs.
1. A and B press their backs together, and each supports the other, pressing backward and upward, as they rise from the floor.

NOTE:
If floor is not carpeted, wear ripple- or other rubber-soled shoes for traction.

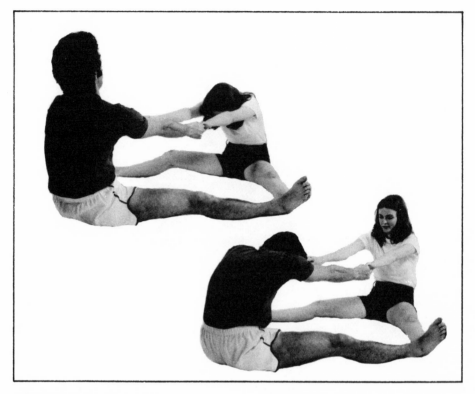

GRANDPA'S ROCKER

GOALS:
Slim shoulders, strengthen back.

START:
A and B sit on the floor, facing each other, the legs apart and feet touching. Each extends arms forward, fingers curled. A extends arms, palms up, B, palms down. B's fingers hook into A's fingers (or they clasp each other's wrists).

1. The partners now rock gently backward and forward, contracting abdominal and back muscles and keeping the rib cage lifted.
TIME:
Thirty seconds.

PAUSGYMNASTIK (OFFICE EXERCISE BREAKS)

The battle of workers' stress and fatigue is being won quickly in Sweden by the introduction of a 15-minute pausgymnastik, or office exercise break.

Confinement to a desk or working in a small area in one position for long periods can result in indifferent work habits and will also cause acute pain in the back and neck muscles and swelling, due to loss of circulation, in the legs and feet.

The following exercises, assembled by the noted Swedish ergonomist Valborg Gisecke, are designed to improve circulation and to help revitalize the worker so that he or she functions more efficiently. They are planned to be particularly useful at conferences or to provide a change of pace for office personnel who sit long periods.

Get up for your exercise break the very first moment your bones cry out for relaxation. Kick off your shoes. Remove restrictive jackets or jewelry. Stand away from your desk and chair, typewriter or office machine, allowing space for free body movement. Open a window if possible, and if a radio or tape or record player is available for music, all the better.

Exercise in a group or alone—but exercise!

1. JOG: Do this lightly in place, alternately lifting right and left heels, for 30 seconds. Then change to light running in place with arms relaxed and moving naturally, for 30 seconds.

2. STRETCH AND YAWN: Stretch arms up along your sides and above your head. Rise on your toes, and reach for the ceiling. Yawn. Let your arms fall limply to the sides. Shake your shoulders. Repeat stretch and yawn for one minute.

3. SHOULDER ROLL: Rotate shoulders back, down, and forward, keeping arms relaxed. After several rolls, shake shoulders, and continue, alternately rolling and shaking for a full minute.

4. SIDE BENDS: Stand, feet apart. Bend sideways to the left, and bounce gently four times. Return to standing position and repeat to

the right. Mark rhythm by clapping hands behind you as you return to an upright position: Bend, bounce, bounce, bounce, bounce, clap!

5. SIDE TURNS: Stand, legs apart, elbows bent. Place fingertips on shoulders. Turn body to the right; twist harder, and bounce to the right. Now forward, turn body to the left; twist harder, and bounce to the left. Forward again, and repeat six times. Keep your eyes focused on one spot in front of you, to avoid getting dizzy. Set rhythm for the exercise by snapping your fingers at every second, harder twist.

6. BACKBENDS: Stand, legs apart, hands clasped in front. Bend forward from the waist, first over the left leg and straighten, then over the right leg and straighten. Keep neck and arms loose.

7. NECK BENDS: Stand with legs wide apart, arms relaxed at sides. Bend head slowly to the left, then slowly to the right. Repeat alternately left and right several times. Drop head back, forward, right, back, left, and around to the front.

8. HOP AND JOG: Hop alternately twice on the left foot and twice on the right, raising the opposite knee. Finish with a light jog.

9. STRETCH AND RELAX: Stand, feet together, arms and hands relaxed at the sides. Swing arms forward and up, and let them pull gently back, behind head. Let arms fall heavily downward, as you knee-dip slightly. Inhale as your arms move forward and upward; exhale as your arms move downward.

RULES FOR OFFICE WORKERS

1. Don't cross your legs for long periods. Crossing your legs is equivalent to wearing tight garters.
2. Don't sit for more than an hour without getting up and moving.
3. Don't sit if you can stand. Stand to answer the telephone; stand

to refer to the filing cabinet, even if you can reach the files by spinning about in your chair.

4. When rising from your chair, use your back leg as a lever to bring you up.

5. Try to get a chair that allows variations in sitting positions and leg movement.

HUSMORGYMNASTIKEN
(FITNESS FOR HOUSEWIVES, SWEDISH STYLE)

Husmorgymnastiken, or housewives gymnastics, first began in Sweden in 1942. Today this physical-fitness program has more than 100,000 members divided into more than 2,000 groups, which meet in 1,500 urban and rural locations in Sweden.

The housewives' program includes a modified form of physical training for girls and women, usually performed with music. Its aims: to provide exercise in a pleasant atmosphere, to keep the body supple, teach correct breathing techniques, relax tension, and strengthen all parts of the body.

Begin your exercise routine as soon as you rise in the morning or with a group of neighbors in midmorning, as the ladies do in Sweden. Better still, start your own husmorgymnastiken right here, in the U.S.A.!

Turn on the radio or tape or record player and begin:

1. BREATHING EXERCISE: Lie on your back. (Use a slantboard if you have one.) Place your feet on the rung of a chair, and turn them outward to ease the blood flow back to the heart from the legs and feet. Put your hand on your abdomen, just below the rib cage. Feel it rise when you inhale and fall when you exhale. The shoulders should not lift if you are breathing properly. Practice this exercise faithfully; then repeat it throughout the exercise program and throughout the day, sitting or standing.

2. BODY STRETCH: Remain lying on your back. Extend your arms overhead. Stretch your entire body langorously, from the

crown of your head and the tips of your fingers to your toes. Bend your knees to your abdomen, and relax.

3. SIT-UPS: Remain lying on your back, knees bent. Slowly rise to a sitting position. Then return slowly to a lying position, curving your back, vertebra by vertebra, until supine. *Repeat breathing exercise.*

4. OFF-THE-FLOOR LIFT: Turn over, face down. Place your hands on the floor, palms down, beneath the shoulders. Push up on your arms, bending back the upper part of your body. Lower yourself to the floor. Repeat movement. Then lift your left leg as far as you can. Lower left leg. Lift your right leg as far as you can. Lower it. Alternate lifts with legs three times. *Repeat breathing exercise.*

5. SHOULDER SHRUGS: Raise your shoulders, and lower them. Repeat. Rotate shoulders by bringing them up, back, down, and forward twice. *Repeat breathing exercise, standing.*

6. ARM CIRCLES: Extend arms forward, shoulder level. Swing arms in a wide circle, up, back, around, and down, four times. *Repeat breathing exercise.*

7. SIDE TURNS: Stand with your legs wide apart, arms at your sides. Swing both arms from the left hip to the right and back again, keeping hips forward, twisting only from the waist. Repeat ten times. *Repeat breathing exercise.*

8. JOGGING: Jog, or walk in place, lifting your knees high, for one minute. Then hop or walk on each leg, lifting the knees high and swing your arms freely, bringing the opposite arm forward with each knee lift. *Repeat breathing exercise.*

9. SLOW BENDS: Stand with legs about 15 inches apart. Bend forward slowly, starting from the head and following through with the rest of the body. Flex your knees a little until your arms hang

limply almost to the floor. Slowly rise, beginning at the base of the spine, and lift, vertebra by vertebra, unbending the head last, until you are upright. *Repeat breathing exercise.*

10. ARM STRETCH: Stand with feet shoulders' width apart, and stretch arms above your head. Stretch up hard with the left arm so that you feel the stretch all along your side. Repeat with the right arm. Then extend arms to the sides, shoulder level, and stretch to the sides with both arms, twice. *Repeat breathing exercise.*

11. SIDE BENDS: Stand with legs wide apart. With straightened legs, bend the upper part of the body to the side slightly, stretching upward. If you can, stretch the arms over your head while bending. Otherwise, bend with your arms relaxed at your sides, a less difficult exercise. *Repeat breathing exercise.*

12. HEAD-NECK BENDS: Still standing, relax your head and neck. Bend forward limply, rounding only the upper part of the body. Flex the knees slightly. Roll back up, vertebra by vertebra, bringing the head up last, until you are fully upright. *Repeat breathing exercise.*

MEDELALDERS OCH ALDRE TRAININGSPROGRAM (EXERCISES FOR THE FIFTY-PLUS)

Gymnastics programs for older persons are now nation-wide and serve as a source of encouragement for the elderly who need to stay active both physically and socially. Poor circulation has been improved, and stiffened joints and weak muscles have disappeared.

The following exercises have been modified to fit the needs of the aged and the handicapped, who are cautioned to take frequent rest periods until the exercises can be performed comfortably. They have been approved by members of the medical profession and experts in geriatric research and have been recommended by Dr. Per-Olof Astrand.

• Avoid stretching, jerky movements during the back exercises. People in the middle years should be careful not to strain the body joints. Do not move the joints when they are supporting the body's full weight.
• Try to perform your exercise program at least twice weekly. Optimum, every day.
• Exercise to music you love, for greater enjoyment.
• If cardiovascular strain is possible from jogging or running, don't run, walk. But walk briskly. Do not perform step test in the first exercise. And omit Exercise 7.
• Repeat breathing exercise after every other sequence.

1. HOP, SKIP, OR WALK: Hop in place, keeping both feet together or skip rope, or do step test with a bench or stool eight to 16 inches high. (Remember, the step test exercises the heart and must be performed with restraint. If you have knee-joint problems, or suffer from dizziness, do not do this one.) Step onto the stool, then step off, 20 to 30 times a minute. Work for one minute, rest half a minute, then work another minute. Or walk in place, lifting the knees as high as you can.

2. LEG-BODY LIFTS: Lie face down with a pillow under the abdomen. Extend arms forward, palms down. Lift legs and upper part of body so the pillow supports your weight. Repeat five to 20 times for 30 seconds to two minutes.

3. SHOULDER ROLLS: Stand, legs apart. Bend elbows, and raise them to just below shoulder level, with hands just below armpits. Rotate elbow points five times forward and five times backward. Repeat forward and backward rotation four times, for 30 seconds.

4. ARM SWINGS: Stand with legs wide apart, arms relaxed at sides. Swing arms out and above head, around and down in criss-crossing circles. Circle 20 times, changing direction every five revolutions.

5. LEG-AND-ARM SWINGS: Stand with one hand resting on a support. Swing leg and arm forward and back 20 times, but changing sides every five times. Remember: Swing the left arm back as the left leg comes forward; then the arm swings forward as the leg swings back.

6. HIP ROLLS: Stand with legs shoulders' width apart, hands on hips. Roll hips to the right side, back, around to left, front, and around again five times. Repeat hip roll five times in the other direction, starting the roll to the left.

7. PUSH-UPS: Stretch out on the floor, face down. Place hands, palms down, on the floor directly under shoulders. Keep feet close together. Now push up your body. Try to hold it off the floor, keeping your back perfectly straight, with just hands and toes touching the floor. Do not let your back sag. Bend your arms to lower your body until your chest is within two inches of the floor, with your back still straight. Repeat one or more times, for 30 seconds. If your arms are not yet strong enough for this exercise, rest them on a low box or stool until your arms strengthen.

8. HOP 'N' JOG: Hop in place, with legs together, or jog or walk in place, lifting the knees high, for 30 seconds.

9. HOP, SKIP, STEP: Hop in place, skip rope, do step test, or jog and run in place, or just walk in place, remembering to lift your knees as high as you can.

10. LIE flat on your back on the floor, legs slightly elevated, and rest!

PART IV
A PROGRAM
TO FIGHT FATIGUE

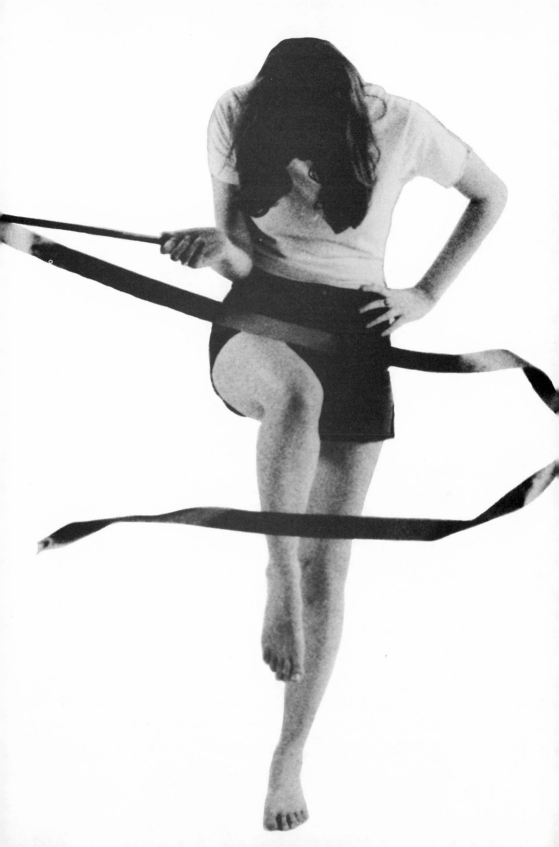

SEVEN

THE BATH

Ah-h-h-h! Peace—it's wonderful! And so is the bath experience if you don't just dunk in and out. Few creature comforts have a greater potential for relaxing and cheering mind and body.

A daily fitness program should include pampering. Shower daily for a quick cleanup, but set aside time to luxuriate in your bath. Create a meaningful bathtime that not only will cleanse your skin and renew its texture, but also will untie all the tangles in your head and body.

YOUR BATH NEEDS

• Two bath pillows provided with small suction cups, one to place behind your head, the other in the small of your back to ease spinal nerve tension.
• A bath tray that extends across the tub to hold herbal eye lotion, gauze pads, creams, nail-grooming accessories, pumice for elbow and foot calluses, and, of course, a book.
• Superfatted soap for all skin types.
• A long-handled bath brush.
• A pinch of borax to soften hard water, or ⅓ of one of the herbal preparations below. Water temperature adjusted to suit your preference. Remember that hot water (98 to 104 degrees or higher) is extremely debilitating, especially to old people.

THE PREPARATION OF HERBS

Herbal preparations do not involve the alchemist's expertise, whatever their extraordinary results.

• An infusion is the liquid resulting from pouring boiling water over crushed, dried or fresh herbs.

Formula:

> 4 heaping tablespoons of dried herb leaves or flowers (Use twice the amount if herbs are fresh).
>
> 2 cups of boiling water (or one cup for stronger infusion).

Place herbs in a glass, china or earthenware bowl. (Do not use metal in any herbal preparation.) Pour boiling water over herbs; cover and let steep for thirty minutes.

PEPPERMINT-AND-LAVENDER BATH OIL. This bath oil softens the skin; unlike many commercial preparations it is water-soluble, and won't leave a residue of film on the tub or you.

Preparation:

2 eggs
1 capsule Vitamin A oil
1/4 teaspoon oil of peppermint
1/4 teaspoon oil of lavender
1 cup sesame oil
1 tablespoon nondetergent
   liquid soap

1/4 cup 70-percent isopropyl
   rubbing alcohol
1/2 cup whole milk
1/2 teaspoon peppermint extract,
   or 1 teaspoon floral cologne

Use only glass or china container in preparation. Place eggs in a quart bowl, and beat to a froth with an electric or rotary beater. Puncture capsule, and drain into eggs. Add the oils, and beat thoroughly. If you are using an electric beater, set it at its lowest speed, and add the soap, drop by drop, beating all the while. Add the alcohol, 1/4 teaspoon at a time, while continuing to beat. Add the milk slowly, and beat thoroughly. Add peppermint extract and stir well. Store in refrigerator in a wide-necked pint jar as it is too thick to pour easily. Add 1/2 cup to your bath water.

BARLEY BATH MIX

Preparation:

2 tablespoons barley flour (obtain from pharmacy)

1 pint cold water

Infusion of 10 ounces dried chamomile

½ teaspoon oil of heliotrope

Mix barley flour with enough of the cold water to make a smooth paste. Add remainder of the pint of cold water, and cook in a double boiler over boiling water for ½ hour. Add chamomile infusion, mix thoroughly. Add oil of heliotrope, and stir until oil is completely absorbed. Add ⅓ to bath water.

BATHS FOR ALL SEASONS

ELDER FLOWER BATH MIX is used as a springtime stimulant for sluggish skins and tired bodies. Add to a full bath:

Infusion of 7 ounces dried elder flowers

3 ounces of dried rosemary

PEPPERMINT SODA BATHS are particularly refreshing in hot weather, and soothing for sunburn and dried skin.

Preparation:

Infusion of 3 ounces dried peppermint

1½ ounces dried spearmint

1 teaspoon oil of peppermint

½ pound of baking soda

Add oil of peppermint to herbal infusion. Add to lukewarm (not hot) bath water when tap is turned on full force. Then add baking soda, and whisk bath water so the soda is fully dissolved.

THE SEA-WATER BATH holds life-giving minerals that are believed to feed the skin during bathtime and soothe rheumatic and arthritic pain. The sea water also acts as a skin detoxicant by inducing perspiration.

Preparation

Add boiling water to cover 1 cup packaged seaweed or seaweed foliage solution available in your local herb shop. Or if you live near the ocean, add the boiling water to 4 cups seaweed washed up on the sand at high tide.

Prepare the seaweed infusion in a glass jar. Cover, and let steep for 1 hour. Strain. Add infusion to your bath water. Don't discard the seaweed! It is used as a massage glove to ease aching joints. And the next time you are at the seashore, don't fail to bottle some sea water in plastic or glass gallon jugs for your home health-spa.

THE SALT WATER BATH RELAXANT is used to provide the same skin-detoxicant action as the Sea-Water Bath. And it will soothe and lull you into a good night's rest.

Preparation:
Add 2 cups of sea salt or kelp (available at herb shop) to 1 quart of boiling water; let stand 15 minutes. Strain if kelp is used. Add ½ teaspoon oil of eucalyptus; stir. Add to bath water.

GOLDEN APRICOT AND ORANGE BLOSSOM OIL BATH will soften and feed coarsened and sallow skin with its oil and vitamin ingredients.

Preparation:

½ cup sesame oil
½ teaspoon oil of apricot
¼ teaspoon oil of orange blossoms
2 capsules Vitamin E oil
1 tablespoon nondetergent oil-based liquid soap

2 tablespoons 70-percent isopropyl rubbing alcohol
¼ cup whole milk
Dash of toilet water or cologne, optional

Combine sesame oil with perfume oils. Puncture capsules and drain into oil mixture. Slowly add soap, while beating with rotary beater. Add alcohol, drop by drop, beating all the while. Slowly add milk in the same fashion. Pour into full bath, and add toilet water or cologne for added fragrance.

LIME FLOWERS AND PEPPERMINT FOOT BATH is believed to have benefits that travel all the way to your head. Improving foot and skin circulation is said to revitalize internal organ circulation, all of which can relieve headaches that may be due to blood congestion.

Preparation:
Infusion of 4 ounces lime flowers
2 ounces peppermint leaves
2 ounces burdock

Fill a plastic bucket with enough hot water (98 to 106 degrees) to immerse feet and calves. Fill another bucket with cool to cold water (55 to 75 degrees). Add herbal infusion to the hot water. If necessary, keep a cool, moist compress on your head to ease congestion. Immerse feet and legs for 10 minutes in the hot herbal bath. Transfer legs and feet to the cool foot bath for 2 minutes, then immerse them again in the herbal-infusion bath. Use contrasting soakings until herbal solution has cooled.

THE SUN BATH should be taken with a protective coating of sesame oil massaged into the skin. Always keep the head covered with a scarf or sun hat. Draw the sun's virtues to your skin slowly. Begin with a 10-minute exposure, and gradually increase sun-bath time to 20 minutes. Follow a sun bath with a lukewarm to cool shower, and apply moisturizer to whole body.

HIMMEL-SOL-OCH-VATTEN BADDRAKT (SKY-SUN-AND-WATER BATH: Fill an outdoor fiberglass pool (made for children or water lillies) with water (or sea water) and add infusion of seaweed. Massage body with sesame oil. Immerse as much of you as will fit into the pool, and let your skin be bathed by the air, sun, and the sea water, while you dream. Your spirits will derive as much from your Himmel-Sol-Och-Vatten Baddrakt as will your body.

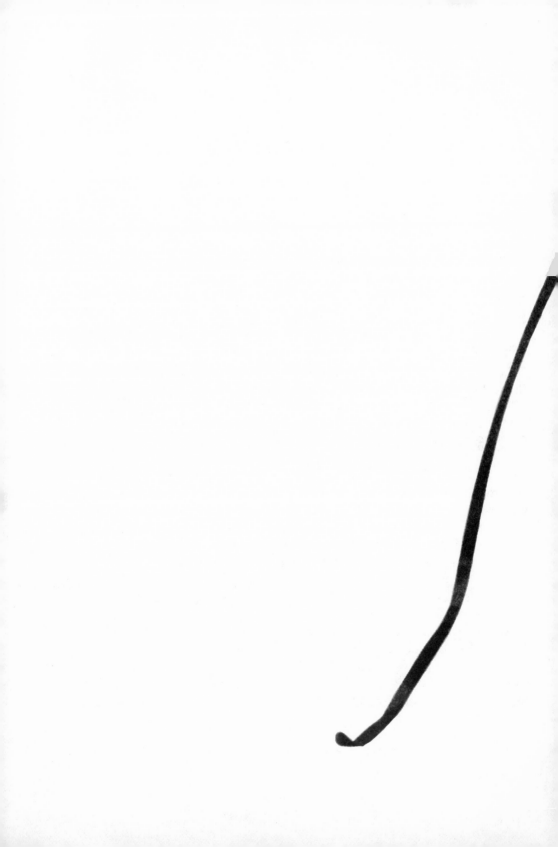

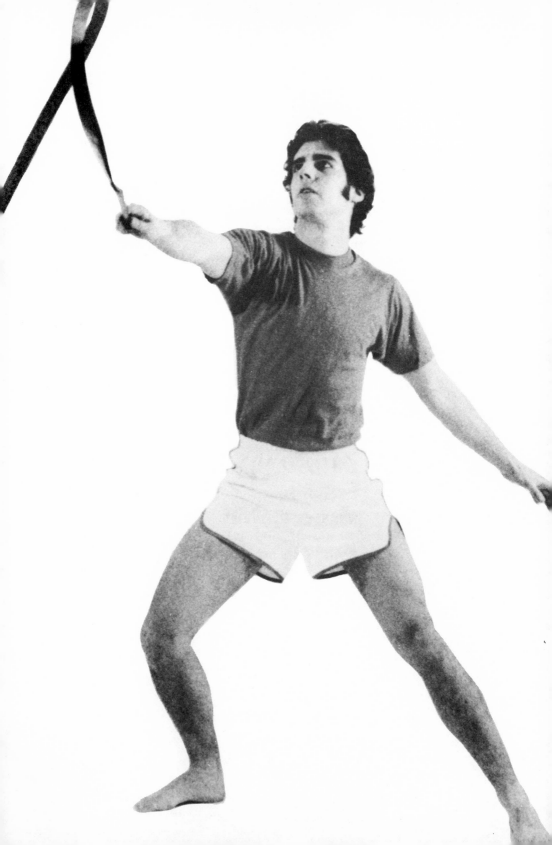

EIGHT

THE WAY TO FIGHT FATIGUE

Certainly the Swedes are mortal. Certainly they get tired and their energy can reach a debilitating low. But what many of them know that we forget is how to save energy, how to bank it and use only as much as is needed—for work, for play, and for sports.

Spending our store of energy over petty annoyances, misplaced objects, irritating associates, or imaginary or exaggerated personal affronts is an extravagance even the wealthiest cannot afford. Anger or frustration can waste precious energy that should be saved for better use.

What inevitably follows when your vitality has been squandered is a state of depression, with its aftermath of anxiety, lethargy, and, often, insomnia. Your appetite may disappear, or you may have an intense and harmful desire to stuff yourself with food.

It is pointless to try to escape the pressures of an urban society. You can't ignore them, hide or run from them; the social pressures will still exist. You can't elude them with pretense that they don't. Nor will wishing erase them. You must encounter them.

But that doesn't mean you must surrender to them.

You can and must insulate yourself against the damage these stresses can cause. You cannot permit them to wreak havoc with your glandular system, subjecting you to the dangers of heart ailments, kidney disfunction, high blood pressure, diabetes, arthritis, allergies, or more and worse.

Were you to look for the villain, you would find that it is tension.

Tension is the culprit. Tension is one of the greatest enemies of longevity. Tension is the monster that breeds anxiety, frustrated rage, ulcers, and utter fatigue. Tension is the parasite that feeds on your life's energy.

Erase the tension, and all other components of that evil family tree will perish.

The store of your energy and endurance can be compared to the number of calories you may or may not spend. There comes a time when your bank may seem empty of those units of energy. Tension has withdrawn it, leaving you at a point of desperation.

Common sense tells you that you must plug the leak. You know that your drive, your energy must be replenished if you are to survive. You feel caged by the pressures and their effect on your whole nervous system, trapped in a maze. You tell yourself, perhaps frantically, "I must relax. I must sleep."

The instincts warning you that only total relaxation and sleep will restore your lost energy are right.

Scientists who have devoted their lives to the problem of combatting fatigue know that the answer to replenishing your store of energy is complete and voluntary physical and mental relaxation resulting from sending the message to the brain: "I am going to relax."

While relaxation may be instinctive with many animals, such as cats, it is not instinctive with adult people. It is necessary for you to acquire physical and mental skill in removing all physical and emotional tension by progressive relaxation of each muscle in turn.

This is not a reflex response. It must be consciously learned, memorized, and made into an acquired habit if you are to triumph over tension and its resultant fatigue.

Come share the secrets of the Royal Swedish Way to fight fatigue:

Every state of nervousness links to the tensing of certain muscles. Your ability to conquer fatigue and renew your reservoir of energy depends on your ability to tense and relax all bodily muscles at will. When you have mastered this technique, you will have taken the first step toward controlling your mental and emotional tensions.

THE TECHNIQUE OF LOCATING YOUR MUSCULAR CONTROL

1. Clench your fist tightly.
   You are now using muscular tension by locating the fist muscles.
2. Slowly relax your fist.
3. Slowly, slowly release your fingers until your hand is limp.
   You have now controlled the tension in your hand by relaxing.
4. Furrow your forehead, drawing your brows together.
   You are now using muscular tension by locating the forehead muscles.
5. Slowly relax your forehead, then your brows.
   You have now controlled the tension in your forehead and brows by relaxing.

Train yourself in this way to tense each muscle, and then let that muscle grow lax, at will, and you will have learned and conquered Muscle Control.

TURNING OFF YOUR MIND

Turn off the visual image of whatever is distressing you. You can accomplish this by imagining yourself and others within your private visual image in a state of complete relaxation. If the cause of your tension or insomnia is concern about whether you can complete a particular task before an early deadline, visualize your hands or body working at that task slowly and still more slowly as if in a slow-motion picture until your body and all its extremities become completely limp. If others are involved in completion of the task on time, imagine them as part of the cast in your dream slowly, slowly yielding, limply, flaccidly.

Think of any element of fatigue as a heavy burden you are carrying on your shoulders. Not until you have freed yourself of this burden can you function efficiently, without tiredness. Fear and worry are at the core of most of the tiredness of the human race.

Often we have in our minds a continuous loop of imaginary terrors far worse than any real penalties we might suffer for failure to meet a deadline, for example. By forcing yourself to think positively, to concentrate on past successes in similar areas and how you achieved them, to know that you can repeat those victories, you may find one way of dropping that burden and destroying that continuous loop of negative thinking.

HOW TO RELAX

One of the first things we are told to do when fatigued is "Relax!" But we know that we cannot achieve physical fitness unless we know HOW to relax. Knowing how to relax is the sought after science:

1. Do not wait until you are almost to the point of no return before you decide that it is time to take a break and relax. Try to take a relaxation break regularly, at approximately the same time each day, depending on your personal requirements and your daily schedule of activities and responsibilities.
2. Find a quiet, darkened room and lie down, or stretch out on a chair. Put your feet up as high as possible.
3. Loosen any restrictive clothing.
4. Let all your muscles go completely limp, your thoughts go to a blank screen.
5. Think now of floating clouds, quiet lakes, all that is slow, serene, relaxing, placid.
6. Mentally seek out the tension in the back of the neck, heighten it voluntarily, and then, consciously, relax it.
7. Now relax your scalp and facial muscles.
8. And your outer and inner throat muscles. This is important because inability to achieve relaxation here is a sure way to transmit tension to others. In extreme shyness, anxiety, anger or tension, the throat tightens, causing the voice to sound harsh, raucous, to rise in pitch or out of control, or even to become inaudible!
9. Relax your shoulder muscles.
10. Release and relax your upper arms, elbows, lower arms.
11. Loosen your wrists, palms, fingers.
12. Then your chest and your abdomen.

13. Next, relax your buttocks and your thighs, front and back.
14. Release any tension in your knees. Let them go limp.
15. Now relax the calves of both legs.
16. Loosen your ankles, the arches of your feet, your toes.
17. With your lips loosely shut, breathe in through the nostrils slowly, deeply.
18. Exhale gently, evenly, letting your breath out through slightly parted lips.

Devote at least 15 minutes, preferably half an hour, to this exercise. Arrange to do it before dinner if you need to call on your energy reserves in the evenings. Try it after lunch if your afternoons are the time for your primary achievements.

If your work is especially tiring physically, here is a variation on the program you might try: Roll up six medium-size towels. Lie on your back. Place one towel behind the neck, one beneath each of your lower legs, bending the knees slightly. Place one in the small of the back and one under each hand, palms down, with arms about eight inches from your sides.

Follow with the program of total, inch-by-inch relaxation.

WARNING SIGNALS

Your eyelids are getting heavy. Unwarranted fears seem to sieze you. Your arms and legs feel heavy, difficult to move. You drop things. You flare up in resentment or unexpectedly feel like crying. Minor annoyances seem magnified in importance beyond what your intelligence tells you is their significance. You start making too many mistakes. Your voice becomes abrasive, and people look at you in puzzlement.

These are just a few of the ways you may recognize physical exhaustion or tension. At the first sign, take immediate, corrective action before your troubles become amplified.

Some nutritionists advise multiple vitamins and mineral capsules taken daily with a supplement of vitamin E. If you plan to go partying, carry vitamin B-complex tablets with you; many believe they replace any depletion of vitamin B caused by alcoholic intake.

Vitamin B, like a well-balanced high-protein diet, helps sustain energy.

• Too much physical exertion? Stop at the first hint of exhaustion unless you are in athletic competition. Lie on your back, or settle back in your chair, drop your head forward, and relax immediately, inch by inch. Then, if possible, take a cat nap.

• Racing about madly? Bring yourself to a screeching halt. Take stock. Where are you going? Why? Is all this urgency necessary? Will this hurry get you there any faster? Even wearing the look of haste can reduce the energy you have in reserve.

• Muscles knotting at the back of your neck, in your legs, abdomen? Heart racing? When the first hint of tension comes on, determinedly make yourself go limp and relax.

• Do ordinary sounds suddenly seem extra loud? Take brief, seven-minute holidays during the day to cut yourself loose. Within your mind, escape to calmness and quiet and make yourself relax.

• You feel a surge of anger, even a justified one. Don't grind your teeth. Work off the rage in the garden, at home scrubbing, scouring, or painting, or play it off, or walk—briskly, breathing in through your nose, lips shut.

• Involved in quibbling arguments? Agree. Nothing hushes a chicken-squabbling debate as abruptly as the magic words, "You're absolutely right." And the quiet that follows is wonderful while you go on to bigger, better things.

• Frustrated to the point of yelling? Go quietly to an empty room, or outdoors if yours isn't a crowded neighborhood, and do just that. Yell. Once. Good and loud. Then relax. (If you haven't started to laugh before the yell is completed, permit yourself to do so once it's out of your system. Remember, laughter is tension's greatest antidote and a great way to sidestep ulcers and heart attacks.)

• Overwhelmed by the number of today's chores and the limited time available? Write down the things you must do in the order of their importance and urgency. Then relax, and tackle them one at a time.

• Feeling closed in on by your living environment? Reexamine it. Is ventilation poor? Lighting inadequate? Temperature too hot or too cold? Noise nerve shattering? Once you identify what's wrong, correction is easier to accomplish. If building insulation is insufficient, the Swedish people have learned to insulate against noise and oppressive heat and cold with draperies, fabric wall hangings, and walls of books.

• Feeling particularly low? Take the Swedish cue. Go cycling, boating, or picnicking. Make plans for a pleasant evening with some person or people you especially like. Perhaps a midnight smorgasbord. Or on a white winter night, gather with friends over a bowl of *glog,* or *glywine.*

• Does tiredness cling to your bones day after day, week after week? There could be a physical reason. Best see your doctor for an allover checkup. The trouble may be caused by something as simple as your need for a tonic or new glasses or better-fitting shoes that won't throw your back out of alignment.

• Do you brood over your yesterdays? Don't let that be the cause of fatigue. Sleep it off; then laugh it off. Tomorrow is another day, and you know better than ever to do *that* again, whatever it was you were castigating yourself for.

• Worrying about what might happen tomorrow? May as well stop. Chances are it won't. Fear and worry can bring on the same life-draining fatigue as can senseless, prolonged running.

• Your desk or dresser cluttered or messy and bothering you? Get a large carton, label it "Clutter," and brush everything into it.

• Bored? Take a break from the day's routine or change your work pace. A new place to lunch, a new hat, even a new route on your walk to work can be energizing.

• Fear or worry causing your fatigue? Talk it out with a good friend, a trusted clergyman or if you fear a possible illness, your family doctor. Really, you're not alone in facing your problems, but the corrective action, whether it be seeking counsel or changing an attitude, must be taken by you.

SITTING EXERCISES

Many peope whose work requires them to sit for prolonged periods often feel their bones crying out for comfort. Here are some Royal Swedish stretching and relaxation exercises that help sitters.

1. Neck Release: Sit still. Pull in your stomach muscles, and let your head flop and circle slowly three times to the right, and three times to the left.

2. Shoulder Circle: Still sitting tall, with rib cage lifted, lift your shoulders high toward your ears, then roll them back, down and up in complete circles, eight times.

3. Arm Roll: Stretch your arms out to the sides, and circle them back, down, and up, ten times.

4. Wrist and Hand Roll: Bend elbows, touching your sides. Circle wrists ten times. Clench fists; open and stretch fingers. Repeat ten times.

5. Leg Exercise: Contract and relax your leg muscles. This improves circulation and helps the blood flow back to the heart. It lessens leg and ankle swellings. Repeat ten times.

Then relax, inch by inch, still sitting at your desk with your head dropped forward or back.

Fatigue and the tension that helps bring it on are your enemies. But if you follow the Royal Swedish Way of combatting them they can never take control of you and you will either preserve your reservoir of energy so you can use it wisely and well or master the art of restoration and replenishment of the drive that can help you achieve happiness and your goals.

PART V
DIET PLANS AND RECIPES

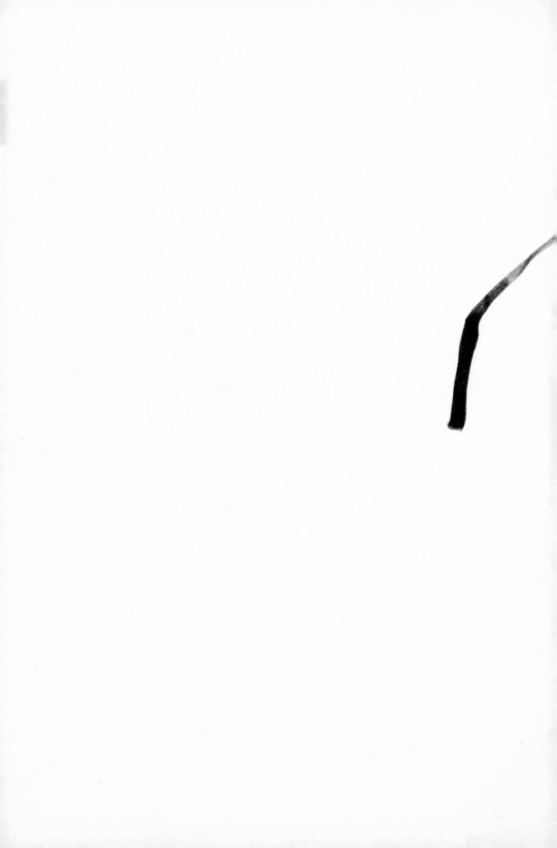

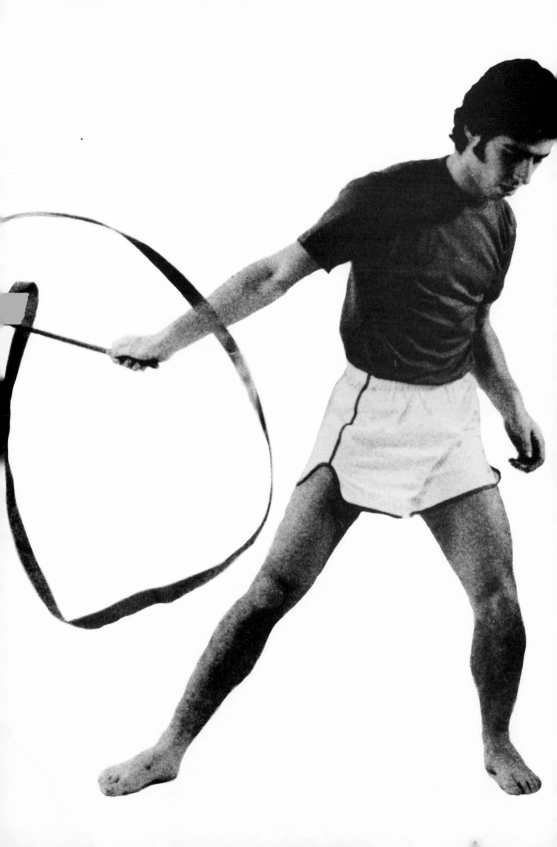

NINE

THE NINE-DAY
1000-CALORIE DIET PLAN

Your body is a negative bank. As in all banks, the more you deposit the fatter your account grows. But your body bank demands that you either refrain from making substantial deposits or spend (burn) all you bank. The penalty for failure? You will grow very, very fat.

Every morsel of candy, cake, and sugar-rich, sticky pastry that you deposit is counterfeit food. These false nutrients contribute nothing to the maintenance of your life. They clog your digestive tract so that layers of ugly fat and the shortening of your lifespan become your punishment for indulging.

Of course food should be enjoyed. But the pleasure of your palate must be guided by the contributions of the six basic nutrient groups: carbohydrates, fats, proteins, minerals, vitamins, and water. These nutrients are needed to give the body its fuel for energy, to build and maintain body tissues, and the enzymes and hormones that are the body's regulators. And they are needed to replace losses that can change the body's whole composition.

Obesity is not a sudden happening. A two-inch slice of cake will add 400 calories and 70 grams of carbohydrates to your food intake. Consuming daily this many more calories and carbohydrates than you can burn through physical activity would result in your gaining 24 pounds of fat in six months, 48 pounds per year, and 240 pounds in five years—if you lived that long! And to burn 400 calories and 70 grams of carbohydrates you would have to swim, nonstop, for more than one hour. It's simply not worth that piece of cake!

Your body furnace first burns the carbohydrates you eat, and only then will it consume those pockets of fat you have stored along your arms, your thighs, your chin and your middle. If you persist in eating more than 60 grams of carbohydrates daily, it never will get around to burning that unwanted body fat for fuel. Until you have reached your weight goal, limit your carbohydrates to 30 grams daily and to only natural sugars found in fruits. After you have achieved your goal, maintain a steady carbohydrate intake of not more than 60 to 70 grams daily.

YOU CAN BE SLIM IF YOU

• Do not skip meals. Being overfed or underfed is destructive to body and mental health. A nutritionally balanced diet will build tissue, not fat, and ensure the healthful functioning of the heart, digestive tract, and complete blood-circulatory system.
• Fasten a warning bell to your cookie jar and refrigerator door.
• Use heavy cooking utensils, preferably with a nonstick finish for sauteing and frying. Then you can cut down on the use of fats in frying.
• Count the calories and carbohydrates you have eaten, and even those you haven't, to boost your morale. But mark in RED letters that the C & C's in candy and pastries turn to fat.
• Exercise regularly while dieting, to strengthen and limber muscles, to aid the circulatory and digestive systems, to tighten skin flab—all of which will lead you to liking yourself.
• Take a multivitamin-plus-mineral capsule daily, but not to replace the nutrients in your daily diet.
• Weigh your foods on a small postal-type scale. Eat only those quantities and foods in your menu program; no less, no more.
• Drink at least eight six-ounce cups of liquid daily. This may include unlimited amounts of beverages. You may have, including tea, skimmed milk, bouillon, noncaloric carbonated beverages, and water. No, liquid will not add to your body weight. Yes, water

will aid in the wash-away process of waste and is necessary for kidney function, circulation and temperature regulation.

• Take bouillon or herb-tea breaks during the day to stave off hunger pangs, to provide energy or restful sleep.

• Weigh yourself, nude, each morning before breakfast. If your scale indicates a weight gain of more than three pounds more than your weight a day or two before, review your food "sintake" during that day, and repent by abstension!

• Think of your diet program from day to day, not week to week. Take one step at a time to reach your weight goal without frustration. Dwelling on innumerable weeks and months would make your desired self-image seem an impossible fantasy—but this is destructive negativism. IF YOU TRULY WANT TO LOSE WEIGHT, YOU CAN.

THE ONE-DAY DETOXIFICATION DIET

Every diet should begin with a thorough inner cleansing without the abrasive action of commercial laxatives. Oranges, lemons, and grapefruit are nature's body-brooms. The natural acids of these citrus fruits are nature's enemies of harmful intestinal bacteria.

Each living organism needs rest. So does your digestive tract. Unlike solid foods, citrus juices, while stimulating the activity of the gastric glands, do not need the digestion of solid-food bulk. They go about their work of cleansing and strengthening while the digestive tract receives needed surcease from action.

Apples create natural bulk, which gently activates the intestines. The combination of the mineral and vitamin content of citrus fruits and apples and the minerals and laxative properties of blackstrap molasses works to provide the food and cleansing action needed in your detoxification diet.

Preparation of One-Day Detoxicant Diet

½ cup orange juice
¼ cup grapefruit juice
  (unsweetened)

1¾ cups lemon juice
1¼ cups blackstrap molasses

Blend all ingredients thoroughly. Every two hours during the day, pour ¾ cup of the citrus-and-molasses beverage into an 8-ounce glass; fill with water to 8 ounces; drink slowly. Keep beverage refrigerated. Twice during the day, slowly chew half an apple. If you feel that further cleansing is needed, this detoxification beverage may be repeated.

Follow the Detoxification Diet with the addition of those nutrients in your menus that will provide you with the vitamins and minerals essential for the preservation of health and good spirits.

DIET PLANNING

Before you follow the Royal Swedish diet, show the plan to your own doctor and get his approval.

FREE FOODS: VEGETABLES: Eat all you desire, cooked or raw; preferably raw.

all green-leafy vegetables	peppers (green or red)
asparagus	pimento
bean sprouts	radishes (all types)
cabbage	rhubarb
cauliflower	spinach
celery	squash (summer squash
cucumber	or zucchini)
endive	turnip greens
mushrooms	watercress
parsley	

LIMITED VEGETABLES: Limit servings to 5 ounces each.

artichokes	parsnips
beets	peas
broccoli	pickles
brussels sprouts	pumpkin
carrots	sauerkraut
Chinese vegetables	scallions
eggplant	squash (acorn)
okra	tomatoes
onions	turnips

FRUITS
Eat daily 1 citrus fruit and 2 other fruits or ¾ cup berries in season, except fruits particularly high in carbohydrates—namely, bananas, Bing cherries, watermelon. Canned fruits must be prepared without sugar added.

FISH
Eat at least 5 or 6 servings weekly. Canned fish must be prepared with water or rinsed of excessive oils. Serve fish broiled, poached in bouillon or skimmed milk, or baked.

MEATS
Eat weekly 1 serving of liver and 3 meals with lean meat, broiled or roasted or sauteed in bouillon.
all beef cuts (lean or with fat trimmed)
lamb (baked, broiled, or roasted, medium rare)
poultry (baked, broiled, or roasted; serve without skin)
veal (baked, broiled, or roasted, medium rare)

DAIRY PRODUCTS
Eat not more than 6 eggs weekly, boiled, poached, or fried in a nonstick heavy pan or a skillet sprayed with nonstick lecithin. You may vary your diet with these dairy substitutions:

1 egg or:
> 3 ounces hard cheese made with skimmed milk
> 3 tablespoons imitation cream cheese
> 3 ounces uncreamed cottage cheese
> 3 ounces farmer cheese
> 3 ounces pot cheese
> 3 ounces ricotta cheese
> 8 ounces skimmed milk or fat-free yogurt, which may be seasoned with extract flavoring and a sugar substitute
> 1 tablespoon butter or 2 tablespoons imitation margarine

BREADS
Enriched protein breads made with unbleached flour or Swedish crispbreads in brown, golden, light, or seasoned-rye types.

BEVERAGES

Drink 2 8-ounce glasses of skimmed milk or milk made with dry milk powder or 1 glass of skimmed evaporated milk daily. Do not drink more than 2 cups of coffee daily. Teas of all types (except herb teas) should not exceed 4 cups daily. The following beverages may be taken in unlimited quantity:

bouillon
herb teas
noncaloric carbonated beverages, including club soda

Preparation of herb teas:
Use only glass or china in herbal-tea (or infusion) preparation.
Dried-herb teas: Use 1 tablespoon for each cup of boiling
    water.
Fresh-herb teas: Use 3 tablespoons, minced, for each cup.
Pour boiling water over the herbs; put a lid on the teapot or a
    saucer over the cup, and steep for 10 minutes. Strain and
    pour. *Skol!*
Herbs are delicious, especially with a squirt of lemon or orange juice.

FREE FOODS:

Salad Dressings, Sauces, and Seasonings: Optional, unlimited choices.

bouillon cubes or granules
catsup (dietetic only)
clam broth or juice
extracts (pure or imitation flavoring)
gelatin (unflavored only)
herbs
horseradish (white or red)
lemon juice
mayonnaise (dietetic only)
mustard
paprika
pepper
salad dressings (dietetic only)
salt (plain, celery, garlic, onion, seasoned, and butter-flavored)
soy sauce
spices
sugar substitute (granulated or liquid)
vegetable powders (garlic, onion)
vinegar (plain, cider, or wine)
Worcestershire sauce

OFF-LIMIT FOODS:
alcoholic beverages (including beer)
bacon
black-eyed peas
bread products (except those permitted), including biscuits, muffins, rolls
butter or margarine
candied fruits
candy
catsup (nondietetic)
corn
cowpeas
cream cheese (nondietetic)
dried fruits
fruits with excessive carbohydrates: bananas, cherries, coconut, figs, mangoes, papayas, persimmons, watermelon
gelatin desserts (nondietetic)
mayonnaise (nondietetic)
meats (luncheon varieties)
nuts
oils in excess of 1 tablespoon daily
pancakes
pastries (cake, cookies, pies, tarts)
peanut butter
pickled fruits
popcorn
pork
potato chips
pretzels
puddings
rice
salad dressings (nondietetic)
sardines
smoked fish
smoked meats
sodas (nondietetic), fruit punch
spaghetti, macaroni, noodles
sugar (brown, raw, and white)
syrups (all types)

THE NINE-DAY 1000-CALORIE DIET PLAN
FOR QUICK WEIGHT LOSS

Optional: Sugar substitute and a dash of skimmed milk with tea or coffee.

The diet recipes referred to here appear in Chapter 11.

FIRST DAY

BREAKFAST
4 ounces orange juice with 4 ounces hot water
1 egg, poached or boiled
1 slice protein-bread toast
1 pat imitation margarine
Tea or coffee

LUNCHEON
5 ounces white chicken or dark turkey meat
4 wedges raw tomato on lettuce leaves
½ cup low-calorie canned apricots
8 ounces skimmed milk

MIDAFTERNOON: 1 cup bouillon with 1 slice Swedish crisp-
    bread

DINNER
5 ounces ground lean beef, broiled
½ cup string beans
1 wedge lettuce with low-calorie salad dressing
½ cup fresh-fruit salad

SECOND DAY

BREAKFAST
½ grapefruit
3 ounces melted cheese on
   1 slice protein-bread toast
1 pat imitation margarine
Herb tea or coffee

MIDMORNING: Cup of herb tea with dash of lemon

LUNCHEON
2 broiled lamb chops (with fat trimmed)
5 asparagus stalks
½ cup cauliflower
½ cup apple and pineapple chunks (fresh or canned, water-
   packed)
8 ounces skimmed milk

MIDAFTERNOON: 1 medium-size fruit or ½ cup berries in
   season

DINNER
5 ounces fish fillet poached in bouillon with dehydrated chives
½ cup chopped spinach flavored with butter salt
½ cup summer squash or carrots
1 cup green salad: lettuce, cucumber wedges, radishes, raw-
   cauliflower crumbs
8 ounces skimmed milk

THIRD DAY

BREAKFAST
½ cantaloupe
1 egg fried in nonstick or lecithin-sprayed skillet
1 pat imitation margarine
Tea or coffee

LUNCHEON
6 ounces tomato juice with a dash of lime
Crab flakes with celery, endive, and cucumber cubes, with 1
   teaspoon Diet Mayonnaise, on lettuce leaves
1 slice Swedish crispbread
8 ounces skimmed milk

DINNER
5 ounces broiled tenderloin steak (lean)
½ cup zucchini sauteed in diet margarine
½ cup carrots (raw or boiled)
¾ cup noncaloric gelatin dessert
8 ounces skimmed milk

EVENING: Herb tea and 1 pear

FOURTH DAY

BREAKFAST
½ grapefruit
¾ cup nonsweetened cereal
8 ounces skimmed milk
Tea or coffee

LUNCHEON
¾ cup skimmed-milk cottage cheese
½ cup berries in season
1 slice whole-wheat bread
Herb tea or coffee

MIDAFTERNOON: Bouillon or herb tea and choice of fruit
(fresh)

DINNER
5 ounces tomato juice with dash of lemon juice
6 ounces baked trout, prepared with 1 tablespoon oil
5 ounces calves' liver, sauteed in 1 tablespoon oil
½ cup green beans
Salad greens with cucumber quarters and tomato wedges
1 tablespoon Diet Salad Dressing
1 orange and 1 apple, pared and sliced in fruit cup with berry
juice
Herb tea or coffee

EVENING: 8 ounces skimmed milk

FIFTH DAY

BREAKFAST
4 ounces orange juice in 4 ounces hot water
1 egg, scrambled with 1 tablespoon ham bits (prepare in non-stick or lecithin-sprayed skillet)
1 slice Swedish crispbread
1 tablespoon diet margarine
Tea or coffee

MIDMORNING: 8 ounces skimmed milk

LUNCHEON
4 ounces grapefruit juice
Chef's salad: chicken or turkey strips, greens, radishes, 4 tomato wedges, cucumber slices, endive, 4 green-scallion stalks, chopped
Diet Creamy Salad Dressing
Choice of fruit
Tea or coffee

MIDAFTERNOON: Choice of fruit

DINNER
4 ounces tomato juice
6 ounces turbot fillet, poached in bouillon
¾ cup broccoli flowerets
½ cup beets
¾ cup shredded cabbage and green pepper, with 1 teaspoon Diet Mayonnaise
1 apple, baked in noncaloric cherry soda
Tea or coffee

EVENING: 8 ounces skimmed milk

SIXTH DAY

BREAKFAST
½ cantaloupe
½ cup skimmed-milk cottage cheese, seasoned with cinnamon
    and sugar substitute, broiled on 1 slice protein-bread toast
Herb tea of coffee

MIDMORNING: 8 ounces skimmed milk

LUNCHEON
5 ounces canned salmon, water packed, with 5 onion rings
    (raw)
½ cup chopped spinach
2 tomato halves, broiled with 1 teaspoon diet margarine
1 slice Swedish crispbread
1 apple
Herb tea or coffee

MIDAFTERNOON: Choice of fruit

DINNER
Bouillon, with sliced mushrooms
5 ounces roast chicken (without skin)
½ cup steamed carrots
Spinach-and-pineapple salad: raw baby spinach leaves with ½
    cup pineapple chunks, Diet Salad Dressing
Noncaloric-gelatin mold
Herb tea or coffee

EVENING: 8 ounces skimmed milk

SEVENTH DAY

BREAKFAST
2-inch slice honeydew melon
1 poached egg, served on 1 thin ham slice on 1 slice whole-
grain toast
Tea or coffee

MIDMORNING: 8 ounces skimmed milk

LUNCHEON
6 ounces tomato juice
5 ounces fresh shrimp
Endive-and-cucumber salad, garnished with 2 halved ripe
olives
3/4 cup assorted berries in season
1 slice Swedish crispbread
1 pat diet margarine
Herb tea or coffee

DINNER
2 veal chops, broiled or baked in aluminum foil with 1 teaspoon
sesame oil
1/2 cup steamed broccoli
1/2 cup cauliflower
Raw-spinach salad: young spinach leaves, 1/4 cup chopped
scallion stalks, 3 sliced radishes
1 tablespoon Diet Salad Dressing
1 cup cubed cantaloupe and berries in season
Herb tea or coffee

EVENING: 8 ounces skimmed milk

EIGHTH DAY

BREAKFAST
½ grapefruit
1 egg, scrambled with 1 teaspoon hard yellow cheese
1 slice Swedish crispbread
1 pat diet margarine
Tea or coffee

MIDMORNING: Choice of fruit or ¾ cup berries in season

LUNCHEON
5 ounces sliced pot roast (hot or cold)
2 tomato halves, broiled with diet margarine and garnished with
    1 teaspoon chopped chives
½ cup chopped spinach
1 sliced whole-grain toast or 1 slice Swedish crispbread
½ grapefruit
Tea or coffee

MIDAFTERNOON: 8 ounces skimmed milk

DINNER
5 ounces turbot fillet, broiled
5 stalks asparagus (steamed)
¾ cup tomato aspic (unflavored gelatin, tomato juice, with ½
    cup thinly sliced celery added after aspic has cooled, but has
    not set)
Choice of fruit in season
Tea or coffee

EVENING: 8 ounces skimmed milk

NINTH DAY

BREAKFAST
4 ounces orange juice in 4 ounces hot water
3 ounces melted cheese on 1 slice whole-wheat toast ("buttered" with 1 pat diet margarine)

MIDMORNING: 8 ounces skimmed milk

LUNCHEON
4 ounces tomato juice
Cottage-cheese garden salad (¾ cup skimmed-milk cottage cheese, 1 tablespoon chopped radishes, 1 tablespoon chopped celery, 1 teaspoon chopped scallion stalks), on lettuce leaves
Low-calorie-gelatin mold with 2 tablespoons blueberries
Tea or coffee

MIDAFTERNOON: Bouillon with 1 slice Swedish crispbread

DINNER
5 ounces lean roast lamb
1 teaspoon dietetic mint jelly
½ cup baked zucchini
½ cup baby carrots, steamed with ½ teaspoon dehydrated mint leaves
3 celery stalks (raw)
2 canned water-packed peach halves, topped with ½ teaspoon dietetic jelly in each peach
Herb tea or coffee

EVENING: 8 ounces skimmed milk

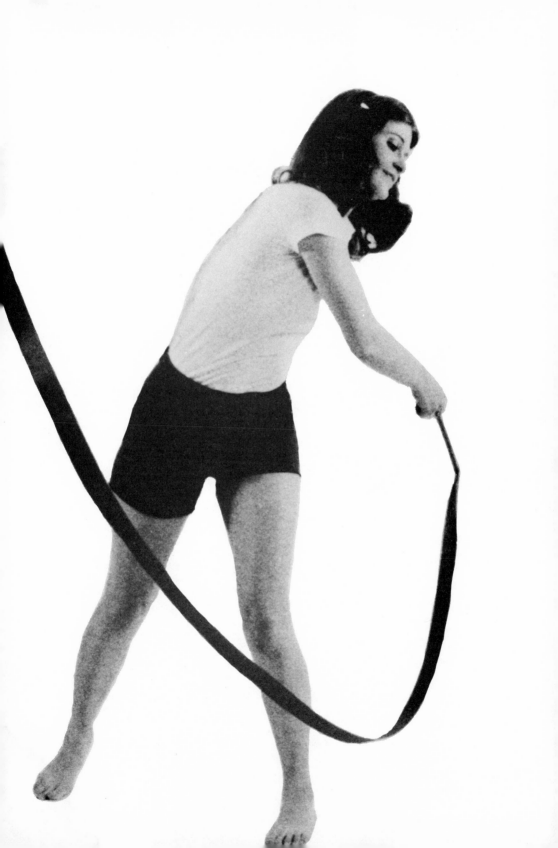

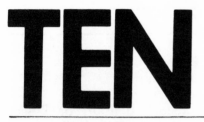

TEN

THE 60-DAY
FOLLOW-UP PROGRAM

Lots of people find taking weight off isn't half as hard as keeping it off. With the Royal Swedish program for exercise and the new buoyancy you will derive from daily exercise the Swedish way, chances are you won't have any trouble staying slim. But do weigh yourself daily; that is very important at this time. If you go up take it right off, and keep it off with the 1200-calorie 60-day follow-up diet described below in a weekly plan.

If you have children or teenagers interested in dieting, the follow-up diet is a moderate program that might be just right. Check it out with your family doctor before applying it to the whole family, however, and browse in the Appendix section at the back of the book. Here you will find additional ideas and information on nutrition for special age groups, and the amount of calories used by various work groups daily.

If, or when, you switch to the 1200-calorie 60-day follow-up plan, be sure that you keep your nutrient intake balanced.

• Continue taking 1 multi-vitamin-plus-minerals capsule daily.

• Add daily 50 milligrams of vitamin B-6, before meals, to aid the movement of body fluids through the bloodstream.

• Add 3 times daily, before meals, 1 tablespoon lecithin granules, to aid in breaking up of fat deposits into fluids, so the body may rid itself of waste plus inches. Place 1 tablespoon of the lecithin granules in blender with 8 ounces of skimmed milk or juice.

• Take 4 10-grain kelp tablets 3 times daily, after meals, to help stabilize your metabolism.

MONDAY

BREAKFAST
6 ounces orange juice in 2 ounces hot water
2 poached eggs
1 slice enriched bread (made with unbleached flour) or 1 slice
   Swedish crispbread
1 teaspoon butter
Herb tea or coffee

LUNCHEON
½ cup skimmed-milk cottage cheese
Fruit salad: 2 apricot halves; 1 pear diced; 1 apple, diced; and
   ½ cup strawberries, with 1 tablespoon Diet Fruit Salad
   Dressing
1 slice Swedish crispbread
8 ounces skimmed milk

MIDAFTERNOON: 6 ounces skimmed-milk yogurt, flavored
   with a dash of almond extract

DINNER
1 cup tomato juice
4 ounces Diet Crusty Lamb Roast
6 asparagus stalks, with Diet Hollandaise
½ cup steamed cauliflower
¾ cup Diet Strawberry Sherbet
Herb tea or coffee

TUESDAY

BREAKFAST
½ grapefruit
1 slice Diet Egg-Toast, with Diet Maple Syrup
8 ounces skimmed milk

MIDMORNING: Herb tea or coffee

LUNCHEON
Diet Baked Salmon Puff
Assorted salad greens, with Diet Creamy Salad Dressing
Choice of fruit in season
Herb tea or coffee

MIDAFTERNOON: 8 ounces skimmed milk

DINNER
4 ounces clam juice
5 ounces broiled sirloin steak (fat trimmed)
¾ cup cubed crookneck squash (boiled in bouillon, seasoned
    with dash of lemon)
6 large mushroom caps, sauteed in 1 tablespoon oil with ½
    teaspoon lemon juice
1 cup fresh strawberries
Herb tea or coffee

WEDNESDAY

BREAKFAST
4 ounces tomato juice
5 ounces lime-broiled turbot fillet (broil with 1 tablespoon diet
    margarine and ½ teaspoon lime juice)
1 slice Swedish crispbread
Herb tea or coffee

MIDMORNING: 8 ounces skimmed milk

LUNCHEON
1 cup beef bouillon
¾ cup Diet Liver Pate, served on lettuce leaves
4 tomato wedges
1 cup diet canned pears (water packed)
Herb tea or coffee

MIDAFTERNOON: 8 ounces skimmed milk or 5 ounces
    skimmed-milk yogurt

DINNER
½ grapefruit
5 ounces Diet Small Meatballs
¾ cup string beans
½ cup Diet Eggplant Bake
3-inch wedge of Diet Lemon-Cream Pie
Herb tea or coffee

THURSDAY

BREAKFAST
4 ounces orange juice
8 ounces Diet Breakfast Custard
1 slice Swedish crispbread
1 teaspoon butter
Herb tea or coffee

MIDMORNING: Choice of fruit

LUNCH
5 ounces Diet Poached Fillets
3/4 cup chopped spinach, garnished with lemon slice
1/2 cup canned artichoke hearts (heat with a pinch of garlic,
    dash of lemon, and butter-flavored extract)
Diet Apple Turnover
8 ounces skimmed milk

MIDAFTERNOON: 1 cup bouillon, with 1 slice Swedish crisp-
    bread

DINNER
1/2 grapefruit
5 ounces sauteed calves' liver, 1/2 inch thick (use heavy skillet,
    and saute 2 minutes on each side in 1 tablespoon safflower
    oil)
1 onion, sliced and sauteed until golden
1/2 cup sliced beets, seasoned with butter salt
3/4 cup coleslaw with 2 chopped olives, 1 tablespoon skimmed-
    milk yogurt, and 1/2 teaspoon fresh mint
1 cup Diet Pineapple Fluff
Tea or coffee

FRIDAY

BREAKFAST
½ grapefruit
2-egg onion omelet (add 1 teaspoon minced onion, dehydrated or fresh, to beaten eggs; wait 3 minutes before
cooking in heavy, lecithin-sprayed skillet)
1 slice whole-grain toast
1 tablespoon diet margarine
Tea or coffee

MIDMORNING: 8 ounces skimmed milk

LUNCH
4 ounces clam juice
5 ounces crab flakes
Diet Tomato Ring
Celery stalks and cucumber quarters
1 slice Swedish crispbread
Choice of fresh fruit
Herb tea

MIDAFTERNOON: 8 ounces skimmed milk

DINNER
6 ounces baked ham, with diet-packed pineapple slice
½ cup parsnips
½ cup Diet Spiced Cabbage
Diet Almond-Filled Baked Apple, with Diet Lemon-
Custard Sauce
Herb tea or coffee

SATURDAY

BREAKFAST
1 cup cubed canteloupe and whole strawberries or blueberries
1 Diet Breakfast Cheese Pastry
1 teaspoon butter
Tea or coffee

MIDMORNING: 8 ounces skimmed milk or 6 ounces skimmed-milk yogurt

LUNCHEON
6 ounces Diet Meat Loaf in Aspic
Apple-and-chopped-celery salad, with Diet Fruit Salad Dressing,
½ cup frozen peas (boiled 2 minutes only)
1 slice Swedish crispbread
Diet Spice Cupcake
8 ounces skimmed milk

MIDAFTERNOON: 1 cup bouillon

DINNER
6 ounces Diet Poached Fish Fillets
¾ cup steamed broccoli flowerets with Diet Hollandaise
½ cup carrot strips, boiled only until tender with fresh mint, 1 teaspoon brown-sugar substitute, and dash of butter salt
Diet Golden Snow
Herb tea or coffee

SUNDAY

BREAKFAST
6 ounces orange juice
1 egg Benedict (place poached egg on thin ham slice on 1 slice
   protein toast; top with Diet Hollandaise
Tea or coffee

LUNCHEON
4 ounces tomato juice
6 ounces Diet Poached Salmon Aspic
½ cup Chinese peapods
½ cup cauliflower buds (flavored with butter salt)
Diet Whipped Lemon Loaf
Tea or coffee

MIDAFTERNOON: 8 ounces skimmed milk

DINNER
2-inch slice honeydew melon
5 ounces Diet Roast Pork
¾ cup baked zucchini
2 broiled tomato halves, garnished with chopped chives
3-inch slice Diet Cheesecake
Herb tea or coffee

The diet recipes referred to here appear in Chapter 11.

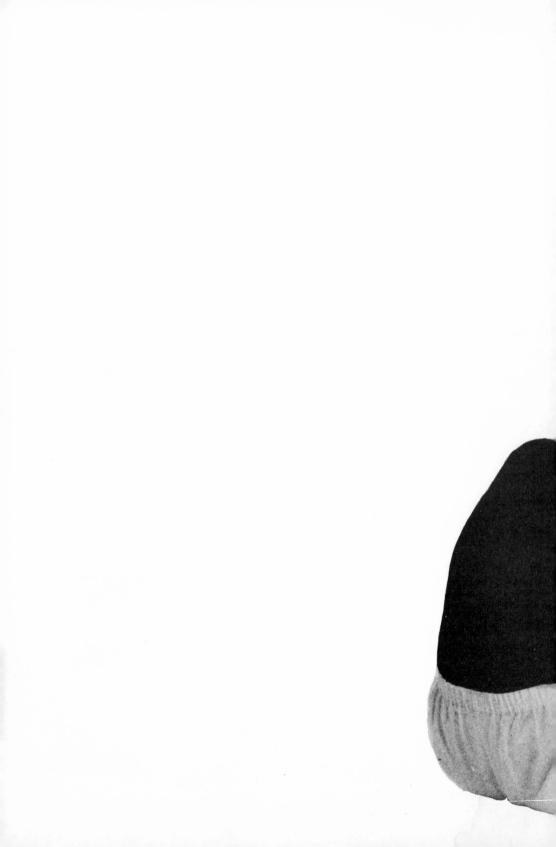

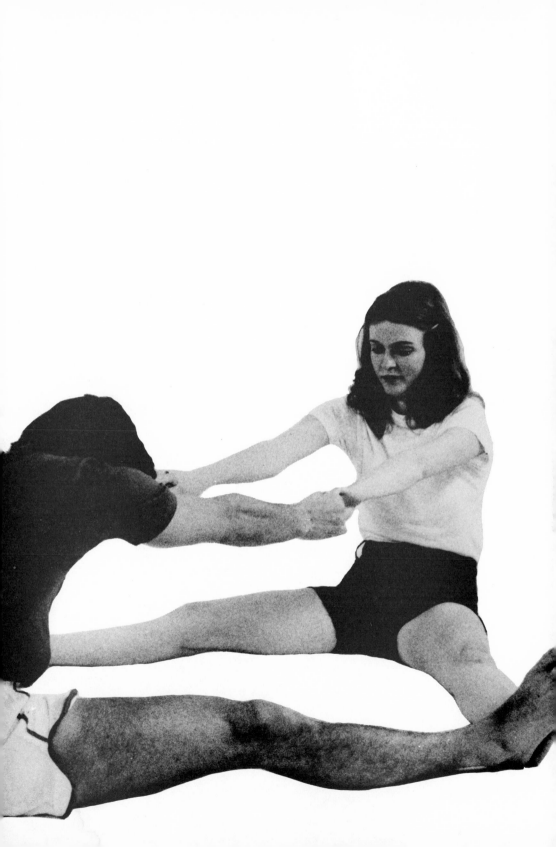

ELEVEN

DIET RECIPES
AND THE DIET SMORGASBORD

The recipes in this chapter are in two groups: the first group includes diet recipes for foods we often use or which are useful as accessories to main dishes, while the second group consists of wonderful smorgasbord dishes from Sweden. The smorgasbord recipes are given in both the original (or nonthinning!) version, and in a diet form. Use the diet form while you are losing weight.

DIET MAYONNAISE

2 raw egg yolks
2 hard-boiled egg yolks
1/4 cup fresh lemon juice
2 cups fat-free yogurt
1 teaspoon herb or seasoned salt

1/2 teaspoon common salt
1/2 teaspoon onion powder
1 teaspoon prepared or dry mustard
Dash white pepper
Dash cayenne (optional)

Beat raw egg yolks, and set aside. Press hard-boiled yolks through a coarse sieve; then blend into a paste with lemon juice. Place yogurt in blender; add hard-boiled yolks and seasonings, and blend to heavy-cream texture. Turn mixture into double-boiler top; add raw yolks, and cook over moderate heat, stirring yolks until blended, then until very thick. If cooking over direct heat, use a heavy saucepan and low heat.

DIET SOUR CREAM

¼ cup skimmed milk   ¼ teaspoon salt
⅔ cup skimmed-milk cottage   Sugar substitute to taste
     cheese   (optional)
1 teaspoon lemon juice

Place all ingredients in blender, and blend at puree speed until mixture reaches sour-cream consistency. If too thin, add a bit more cottage cheese. Add the sugar substitute for use with fruit dishes. VARIATIONS: Add dehydrated minced onion, chopped fresh or dehydrated parsley, chopped mint leaves, chives, and/or other herbs, singly or in combinations.

CREAMY SALAD DRESSING

1 tablespoon Diet Mayon-   1 tablespoon wine vinegar
     naise   Pinch paprika
½ cup skimmed-milk yogurt   Seasoned salt to taste
¼ teaspoon garlic powder   Onion salt to taste
1/8 teaspoon dehydrated   Pepper (optional)
     chives
1/8 teaspoon dehydrated
     parsley

Combine all ingredients in a glass bowl; beat with electric or manual mixer until well combined. Place in a bottle, and refrigerate until needed.

DIET FRUIT SALAD DRESSING

1 cup fresh or canned raspber-   1 cup canned pineapple
     ries or strawberries   (water-packed)
1 tablespoon granulated-sugar   1¼ cup skimmed-milk cottage
     substitute   cheese

Use unsweetened, water-packed berries. Place all ingredients, except cottage cheese, in blender; blend for 10 seconds. Then add cottage cheese, teaspoon by teaspoon, and blend until thick. If dressing is too thin, add a bit more cottage cheese.

DIET SALAD DRESSING

½ cup tomato juice
2 tablespoons cider vinegar
1 tablespoon fresh, or dehydrated, parsley
1 tablespoon fresh, or dehydrated, minced onion
2 tablespoons minced green
pepper

½ cup beef bouillon
½ cup grapefruit juice
Garlic powder or garlic salt to
taste
Dash liquid sugar substitute to
taste

Combine all ingredients in blender, at medium speed, for 20 seconds.

DIET WHIPPED CREAM

4 ounces evaporated skimmed
milk, chilled
1 tablespoon lemon juice

¼ teaspoon unflavored gelatin
Liquid sugar substitute to taste

Be sure milk is well chilled. Add lemon juice and gelatin to milk and whip into stiff peaks. Sweeten to taste.

DIET HOLLANDAISE

2 tablespoons fresh lemon juice
1/8 teaspoon butter extract
½ teaspoon imitation butter
salt
1/8 teaspoon paprika
Dash cayenne

Pinch white pepper (optional)
2 drops yellow vegetable coloring (optional)
1¼ cups skimmed-milk cot-
tage cheese
3 egg yolks, beaten

Place lemon juice, extract, seasonings, and coloring in blender. Turn blender to high speed. After 10 seconds, add cottage cheese gradually; continue blending until mixture is smooth and creamy. Remove from blender, and place in a double-boiler top (but not yet over heat). Stir in beaten egg yolks until thoroughly blended. Place double-boiler top over the bottom, half filled with rapidly boiling water. Cook, stirring constantly with a flexible spatula or wooden spoon, until thick. Do not cook hollandaise over direct heat. Serve hot or cold. Keep refrigerated.

DIET BREAKFAST CHEESE "PASTRY"

2 ounces skimmed cottage cheese
Dash cinnamon

Dash sugar substitute
2 drops vanilla extract
1 slice protein-bread toast

Combine cottage cheese with cinnamon, sugar substitute, and extract. Spoon on toast, and place under broiler until bubbly (about 2 minutes). Makes 1 portion.

DIET APPLE "TURNOVER"

1 apple, peeled, cored, and sliced
1 teaspoon lemon juice
1 teaspoon cinnamon

3 tablespoons water
1 teaspoon sugar substitute
1 slice enriched white bread

Combine apple slices with lemon juice, cinnamon, water, and sugar substitute; cook over medium heat until apple is tender. Cool. Remove crust from bread slice, and roll slice thin. Place half of apple mixture on bread; fold diagonally. Moisten edges, and press them together with aluminum foil. Bake at 325° until crisp, about 35 minutes. Makes 2 portions.

DIET BREAKFAST CUSTARD

1 egg
1 cup skimmed milk
1 teaspoon vanilla

1¼ teaspoons sugar substitute
Cinnamon

Place first 4 ingredients in blender for 5 minutes. Pour mixture into 2 small custard cups. Sprinkle with cinnamon. Place cups in a baking pan with water to cover ¼ inch up sides. Bake at 325° for 45 minutes to 1 hour. Cool, and place in refrigerator to chill. Makes 1 portion.

DIET EGG-TOAST

2 large eggs, beaten
½ cup skimmed milk
Pinch cinnamon
Pinch nutmeg
Pinch salt

1/8 teaspoon vanilla
Liquid sugar substitute equivalent to 1 tablespoon sugar
2 slices enriched white bread
(5/8 inch thick)

Combine all ingredients (except bread) in a deep, wide bowl, beat until thoroughly blended. Add bread, turning each slice until it is well covered. Cover bowl, and let bread soak up egg mixture for 1 hour or longer. Turn bread once or twice, so that slices are evenly saturated. Bake in moderate (350°) oven ½ hour. Serve with Diet Maple Syrup. Makes 2 portions.

DIET MAPLE SYRUP

12 ounces noncaloric cream-
flavored carbonated beverage
1 teaspoon maple extract
1 teaspoon butter-flavored extract

Granulated-sugar substitute
equivalent to 1 tablespoon
sugar

Place all ingredients in a heavy, enamel-coated saucepan, and bring to a boil. Lower heat, and simmer 5 minutes.

DIET LINGONBERRY JAM

4 ounces orange juice
4 ounces cold water
1½ tablespoons unflavored
gelatin
2½ cups lingonberries, stem-

med and rinsed (or other
berries in season)
Granulated-sugar substitute
equivalent to 2 tablespoons
sugar

Place orange juice and water in heavy, enamel-coated saucepan. Add gelatin to soften, and stir until dissolved. Place over heat, and bring to a boil. Add berries and sugar substitute. Stir once; then lower heat to a slow boil. Cook until mixture thickens to a jamlike consistency. Store in a glass or china container in refrigerator.

DIET BAKED SALMON PUFF

4 slices enriched bread, crumbed
2 cups buttermilk
1 teaspoon paprika
½ teaspoon onion salt
Pinch marjoram
Pinch dill weed

1½ tablespoons minced onion (fresh or dehydrated)
4 eggs, separated
1 cup fresh (or canned) sliced mushrooms
8 ounces canned salmon
½ teaspoon cream of tartar

Place in blender bread crumbs, buttermilk, paprika, salt, spices, onion, and egg yolks, and blend for 45 seconds. Combine mushrooms and salmon in a large bowl. Add blender mixture, and mix thoroughly. Place egg whites in a chilled mixing bowl; add cream of tartar, and beat until stiff. Fold into fish mixture. Pour into a lecithin-sprayed baking dish, and bake in a moderate (350°) oven 1 hour. Makes 4 portions.

DIET EGGPLANT BAKE

1 medium eggplant
Dash lemon juice
3 tablespoons minced onion
3 tablespoons sliced mushrooms (fresh or canned)
1 tablespoon diet margarine
1 tablespoon chopped parsley (fresh or dehydrated)

¾ cup protein-bread crumbs
½ teaspoon onion salt
1 egg
4 ounces skimmed-milk mozzarella or ricotta

Cut eggplant in half lengthwise. Place in heavy, enamel-coated saucepan; cover with boiling water, and cook for 15 minutes. Drain. Carefully remove eggplant pulp with a curved grapefruit knife, leaving ½-inch shell. Squirt pulp with lemon juice; chop well and set aside. Saute onion and mushrooms in margarine until onion is golden. Add to eggplant pulp. Add parsley, bread crumbs, salt, and mix thoroughly. Beat egg slightly, and add to mixture, stirring egg throughout eggplant pulp. Fill shells, and place in a baking dish with ¼ cup water. Bake in a moderate (350°) oven 30 minutes. Remove; top with cheese and return to oven until cheese has melted. Makes 4 portions.

DIET POACHED FISH FILLETS

12 ounces fish fillets
½ teaspoon dill weed
1 teaspoon chopped parsley
1 cup chicken bouillon or clam
  broth

1 teaspoon chopped chives
4 lemon wedges
4 parsley sprigs

Place fish in baking dish. Add dill weed and chopped parsley. Pour bouillon over fillets, and sprinkle with chives. Bake in moderate (375°) oven 30 minutes. Serve garnished with lemon wedges and parsley sprigs. Makes 2 servings.

DIET MEAT LOAF IN ASPIC

2 pounds (4 cups) lean ground
  beef or veal
½ cup chopped radish
½ cup chopped celery
¼ cup chopped green pepper
2 tablespoons minced parsley

1 tablespoon minced onion
  (fresh or dehydrated)
3 envelopes unflavored gelatin
1¼ cups cold water
2 cups beef bouillon
Parsley sprigs

Place meat in heavy, nonstick skillet (or coat skillet with lecithin), and brown, stirring constantly to prevent overcooking. Meat should remain tender, not browned to a crisp. Pour off fat. Combine all vegetables, except parsley sprigs, in a large mixing bowl. Moisten gelatin in ¼ cup of the cold water. Bring bouillon to boiling point, and add to gelatin. Add remaining 1 cup cold water. Add meat to hot bouillon-gelatin mixture. Place in a lecithin-sprayed loaf pan, and store in the refrigerator until gelatin is cold, but not set. Add vegetable mixture, and stir until meat and vegetables are thoroughly mixed. Chill in refrigerator until firm. Spoon off fat that has risen to surface of loaf. Turn out of mold; slice, and serve garnished with parsley sprigs. Makes 6 to 8 portions.

DIET GOLDEN SNOW

1½ tablespoons unflavored gelatin
1 cup cold water
½ cup unsweetened canned apricot juice
1 tablespoon liquid sugar substitute
1/8 teaspoon almond extract
6 diet water-packed canned apricots, mashed

2 egg whites
1½ tablespoons fresh lemon juice
¼ teaspoon unflavored gelatin
2 tablespoons evaporated milk, chilled
Mint sprigs

Place 1½ tablespoons gelatin in top of double boiler with the cold water, apricot juice, sugar substitute, and extract. Place over boiling water, and stir until gelatin is thoroughly dissolved. Remove from heat, and beat in the apricots, using an electric or manual mixer. Continue beating until mixture is thick and frothy. Beat egg whites in a separate bowl until stiff; then fold into fruit mixture. Add lemon juice and ¼ teaspoon gelatin to evaporated milk, and beat to whipped-cream consistency. Fold into fruit mixture. Chill. Wreathe each serving with tiny mint sprigs. Makes 6 servings.

DIET SPICE CUPCAKES

6 slices whole-grain-wheat bread, finely crumbed
6 tablespoons brown-sugar substitute
1 cup skimmed-milk powder
1 tablespoon maple flavoring

1/8 teaspoon ginger
1/8 teaspoon cinnamon
1/8 teaspoon ground cloves
1/8 teaspoon rum extract
1/8 teaspoon almond extract
6 eggs, beaten

Place all ingredients in blender for 15 seconds. Spray muffin tins with lecithin, and fill each a little more than half full. Bake in moderate (350°) oven 15 minutes. Makes 18 cupcakes.

DIET WHIPPED LEMON LOAF

4 large eggs, separated
1/4 cup cold water
2 tablespoons fresh lemon juice
1 1/2 teaspoons finely grated lemon peel
3 tablespoons liquid sugar substitute
1 tablespoon pure lemon extract

2 tablespoons vanilla extract
1 teaspoon coconut extract
5 slices enriched white bread (made with unbleached flour)
3/4 cup powdered skimmed milk
1/4 teaspoon cream of tartar

Preheat oven to 350° for 10 minutes. Place egg yolks in blender with water, lemon juice, lemon peel, sugar substitute, and extracts; blend 20 seconds. Toast bread, and crush into fine crumbs. Place crumbs in a large bowl; add skimmed milk, and mix thoroughly. Add mixture in blender to milk-and-crumb mixture; blend thoroughly with an electric or manual beater. (Do not put in blender.) Add cream of tartar to egg whites, and beat until stiff. Fold egg whites throughout batter. Spray a nonstick loaf pan with lecithin. Pour batter into pan; bake approximately 55 minutes. Makes 4 servings.

DIET PINEAPPLE FLUFF

1 fresh pineapple
1/2 cup boiling water
Ice cubes
1 1/2 cups powdered skimmed milk
1/3 cup ice water
1 heaping tablespoon unflavored gelatin

1/4 cup cold water
4 teaspoons liquid sugar substitute
7 teaspoons fresh lemon juice
1/4 cup hot water
1 teaspoon almond extract
1 teaspoon coconut extract
1 teaspoon vanilla extract

Peel, core, and cube pineapple over a large bowl so juice will not be wasted. Place the boiling water in a heavy, enamel-coated saucepan; bring to a boil. Lift pineapple cubes out of bowl (save juice for future use) and into the boiling water. Lower heat; cover, and simmer 1/2 hour. Remove from heat. Mash cooked pineapple.

Put in a chilled bowl resting in a larger bowl of ice cubes, to chill quickly. While fruit is cooling, place milk in a mixing bowl, and beat slowly while gradually adding the ice water. Soften gelatin with the cold water. Add sugar substitute and lemon juice. Add the hot water, to thoroughly dissolve gelatin. After 2 minutes, add gelatin mixture to milk mixture; using electric or manual mixer, beat at fastest speed. Continue beating as you slowly add extracts. When mixture forms stiff peaks, fold in mashed pineapple. Chill thoroughly before serving. Makes 6 to 8 servings.

DIET LEMON-CREAM PIE

2 envelopes unflavored gelatin
1 cup boiling water
½ cup fresh orange juice
2 teaspoons fresh lemon juice

1 cup ricotta
2 tablespoons low-calorie orange marmalade
Meringue pie shell, below

Dissolve gelatin in the boiling water in a quart mixing bowl. Add orange and lemon juices; stir. Chill until firmly jelled. Remove from refrigerator; add ricotta and marmalade, and mix with electric or manual mixer for 3 minutes. Pour into pie shell, and refrigerate until firm.

MERINGUE PIE SHELL

4 egg whites
Pinch salt
1 teaspoon cream of tartar
½ cup powdered skimmed milk

¼ cup granulated-sugar substitute
1 teaspoon vanilla

Preheat oven to 275°. Place egg whites in mixing bowl with salt and cream of tartar; beat until whites stand in peaks. Combine milk and sugar substitute. Slowly, teaspoon by teaspoon, add to egg whites, beating all the while; beat until very stiff. Add vanilla, and beat a few seconds longer. Spread mixture on bottom of well-greased 9-inch pie pan. Bake about 50 minutes, or until crust is light brown and hard to the touch. Makes 6 to 8 servings.

THE SMORGASBORD

One of the great delights of Swedish cooking is the smorgasbord, tempting the palate with an inviting array of beautiful, fragrant, varied food offerings, from which the diner selects his favorites or samples the lot, filling, and usually refilling, his plate as temptations are followed around the table.

The home smorgasbord table may include only six choices or, as in many large restaurants, 60. At first glance, people who have never seen a Swedish smorgasbord are bewildered by the abundance and diversity of the delicacies and uncertain about how and with which of the often unfamiliar dishes to load their plates.

There is a distinct, though unwritten procedure: Each diner goes to the table with a clean plate four times—five if the dessert is not served to you at the table. First, each person selects one or more of the Baltic-herring dishes, which may come in as many as 20 or more shapes and flavors. The second course includes other cold fish dishes, prepared in almost every conceivable way—salmon, lobster, crabmeat, sardines, often eaten with a cucumber salad. The third course includes the cold meat dishes, roast beef, pork, the pates, jellied veal, and various pickled relishes, vegetable salads, and berry sauces.

For the fourth course, once again clean plate in hand, the diner selects, from large containers kept at just the right temperature, hot meat dishes—delectable meatballs in gravy, lamb, veal, ham, beef, and goose roasts, perhaps even roast reindeer.

Here are several traditional Swedish smorgasbord dishes and their Royal Swedish Diet versions—and these are just an introduction to tempt you to make Swedish traditions your own.

In keeping with the smorgasbord ritual, of course we begin with herring.

GOURMET HERRING APPETIZER
Sommarsill
(Traditional)

2 12-ounce jars of matjes-herring fillets in wine sauce

1 cup sour cream or mayonnaise

Dash dill weed

2 hard-cooked eggs

¼ cup chopped pickled red beets

2 tablespoons chopped chives

2 tablespoons chopped cucumber

Slice herring fillets thinly, and place on a rectangular (if available) serving platter. Spread herring with sour cream; sprinkle with dill weed. Separate egg yolks from the whites, and chop both finely. Spoon chopped egg yolks and whites, beets, chives, and cucumber in attractive rows on the fillets. Chill 2 hours before serving. Makes 10-12 servings.

DIET GOURMET HERRING APPETIZER

Use traditional recipe, but substitute Diet Sour Cream or Diet Mayonnaise.

HERRING-AND-APPLE SALAD
Sill-och-Appelsallad
(Traditional)

2 schmalz- or matjes-herring fillets (or 12-ounce jar fillets)
2 small cooked or canned pickled beets
1¼ cups diced cooked potatoes
¾ cup diced pickle
¾ cup peeled, cored, and diced apple
5 tablespoons minced onion

¼ cup liquid from pickled beets
¼ cup mayonnaise
2 tablespoons water
2 tablespoons sugar
Salt and pepper, to taste
2 hard cooked eggs (8 wedges)
Parsley sprigs
¼ teaspoon dill weed
1 cup sour cream

Dice herring. Drain beets, and dice. (Save liquid.) Place all diced ingredients and the onion in a large bowl, and mince so flavors will blend. In a small bowl, combine beet liquid, mayonnaise, water, sugar, and seasonings; blend well. Stir gently into fish mixture. Rinse a 6-cup mold with ice water; dry, and spray with lecithin coating. Pack salad into mold; cover tightly with aluminum foil, or cover with lid. Chill in refrigerator 6 to 8 hours.

When ready to serve, turn mold onto serving platter. Arrange hard-cooked egg wedges around mold, with clusters of parsley and a scattering of dill weed. Serve with sour cream and Swedish crispbread, rye, or pumpernickel. Makes 10-12 servings.

DIET HERRING-AND-APPLE SALAD

Prepare traditional recipe with these exceptions: Omit potatoes; use Diet Mayonnaise and sugar substitute equal to 2 tablespoons sugar.

LOBSTER SALAD
Hummersallad
(Traditional)

1 small head lettuce
2 cups lobster, cut into ½-inch pieces
½ cup crabmeat, flaked
1 cup asparagus, cut into ½-inch pieces
½ cup sliced mushrooms
1 cup baby peas
1 cup thinly sliced celery
¾ cup mayonnaise

½ cup heavy cream, whipped
4 teaspoons fresh lemon juice
½ teaspoon prepared mustard
½ teaspoon paprika
¾ teaspoon curry salt (optional)
1/8 teaspoon savory
1 tablespoon dried dill weed
1 tablespoon minced parsley

Line bowl with lettuce leaves; place next 6 ingredients in layers on the greens, and toss. Mix mayonnaise with whipped cream, and slowly add the seasonings to taste. Then add herbs. Keep dressing of pouring consistency. Pour dressing over salad. Do not toss, but separate salad mixture so dressing reaches throughout. Do not disturb arrangement of lobster and other ingredients or of lettuce. Reserve a little lobster for garnish. Chill in refrigerator for 2 hours. Garnish before serving with a few pieces of the rosiest part of the lobster. Makes 6-8 servings.

DIET LOBSTER SALAD

Prepare traditional recipe, using Diet Mayonnaise and Diet Whipped Cream.

SWEDISH CHICKEN ASPIC
Svenska Hon Saladab
(Traditional)

2 2- to 3-pound broiling chickens
6 cups water
2 medium onions
3 carrots, scraped and sliced
4 celery stalks, cut into 2-inch
   pieces
2 scallions, cut into 2-inch
   pieces
Whole bay leaf
4 whole peppercorns

1 tablespoon garlic salt
1/4 teaspoon garlic powder
2 envelopes unflavored gelatin
4 tablespoons cold water
2 egg whites
1 teaspoon fresh lemon juice
4 celery stalks, diced
10 2-inch-long pimento slivers
6 pimento-stuffed olives, sliced
8 radishes, thinly sliced

Place cleaned and rinsed chickens in a large, heavy enamel-clad, iron or aluminum pot. Add 6 cups water, onions, carrots, 2-inch celery pieces, and seasonings; bring quickly to a boil. Then lower heat to medium; cover, and let simmer 1¼ hours, or until tender. Remove chicken from kettle, and set aside. Strain broth, and discard vegetables. When broth is lukewarm, place in refrigerator or freezer just long enough for fat to congeal on surface. Spoon off and discard fat. Soften gelatin in 4 tablespoons cold water, and stir into 3¾ cups chicken broth. Beat egg whites just until foamy; then stir into broth. Heat slowly over medium heat, stirring constantly, until mixture reaches boiling point. Remove from heat, and cover. After 10 minutes, strain through a fine sieve. Add lemon juice. Return to refrigerator for 5 minutes. Remove from refrigerator, add diced celery, and stir briskly until mixture is slightly thick.

Spray 2-quart mold with lecithin coating. Pour 2 cups of gelatin broth into mold. Line bottom of mold with pimento slivers set lengthwise, 2 inches apart; arrange olive slices between pimento slivers; arrange radish slices around edge. Place in refrigerator for ½ hour, to set slightly.

Slice chicken breasts, and cut rest of chicken into ½-inch chunks. Add 2 cups of remaining gelatin broth to mold. Dip sliced chicken breasts into mold, and arrange around sides of mold. Place chunks in center of mold. Cover tightly, and place in refrigerator to set until firm—5 hours. Makes 10-12 servings.

DIET CHICKEN ASPIC

Use traditional recipe.

SWEDISH LIVER PATE
Leverpastej
(Traditional)

1 pound chicken livers or baby beef liver	2 cups whole milk
1/2 pound pork liver	2 eggs, beaten
Large onion	3/4 teaspoon white pepper
Tart apple, cored and peeled	1 tablespoon salt
4 canned anchovies	1/4 teaspoon nutmeg
3/4 pound chicken fat or butter	1/8 teaspoon rosemary
2 tablespoons flour	1/8 teaspoon ground cloves (optional)

Preheat oven to 350°. Put liver, onion, apple, and anchovies through a meat grinder 3 times. Blend in all but 2 tablespoons chicken fat. Melt remaining fat. Add flour, and cook 2 minutes, stirring constantly. Gradually mix in milk, and cook, stirring until thickened. Add this white sauce to liver mixture. Add beaten eggs and seasonings, and beat until thoroughly blended. Set oven at 350°. Bake in 9-by-5-by-3-inch loaf pan, placed in another pan with 1 inch of water, 1¼ hours. Refrigerate, covered. Use within a week. Makes 12 servings.

DIET LIVER PATE

Prepare traditional recipe, but with these substitutions: Diet margarine instead of butter or chicken fat, skimmed milk or nonfat yogurt instead of whole milk.

POACHED SALMON IN ASPIC
Kokt Lax I Gele
(Traditional)

(Attractive, easy to prepare and to serve)

Court Bouillon	4 or 5 sprigs dill or parsley
1 quart water	2 pounds salmon
3 tablespoons white vinegar	Cucumber slices
1 tablespoon salt	Unflavored gelatin
5 whole allspice	Tomatoes
1 bay leaf	Pickled fresh cucumber
1 small onion, chopped	Mayonnaise
1 small carrot, chopped	

Combine court-bouillon ingredients in skillet. Bring to boil; lower heat;cover, and simmer 15 minutes.

Rinse and clean fish. Wrap in cheesecloth; tie ends so fish can be easily lifted out of pan. Bring Court Bouillon to simmer. Lower salmon into simmering liquid; simmer 25 minutes, or until fish is firm and flaky, not mushy. Remove fish from bouillon. Cool bouillon until cold. Remove fish skin, and place on serving platter. Garnish with cucumber slices.

Strain bouillon through a double layer of cheesecloth. Add 1 envelope unflavored gelatin for each pint of cold liquid. Heat until gelatin is dissolved. Cool until of syrup consistency. Spoon half of gelatin mixture over fish. Place in refrigerator for 15 minutes. Spoon remaining mixture over fish. Chill 15 minutes. Garnish salmon with tomatoes filled with pickled fresh cucumber and with mayonnaise. Makes 10 servings.

JANNSSON'S TEMPTATION
Jannssons Frestelse
(Traditional)

(Very tempting served on smorgasbord or as appetizer)

1 cup sliced onions (1½ onions)

⅓ cup butter or margarine

4 cups peeled raw potatoes cut into very thin strips

1 can Swedish anchovy fillets (about 18 fillets)

1 cup milk

Saute onions in 2 tablespoons of the butter. Butter 1½-quart baking dish. In it, arrange layer of half the potatoes. Spread on onions and anchovy fillets; top with remaining potatoes. Sprinkle 1 tablespoon juice from anchovy can over potatoes, and dot with remaining butter. Add milk, and cover with aluminum foil. Bake in hot (400°) oven 30 minutes. Remove foil; bake 20 minutes longer, or until potatoes are tender and golden. Serve immediately, in baking dish. Makes 4 servings.

WEST COAST SALAD
Vastkustsallad
(Traditional)

(Swedish West Coast, famous for its variety of seafood, has given its name to this unusual and delicious salad. Nothing is set about this salad; you can add or deduct ingredients to taste or budget, but mushrooms lose flavor and crispness if marinated too long. In Sweden this salad is served with buttered toast, as an appetizer.)

Salad

½ pound fresh mushrooms
Lemon juice
1 pound cooked shrimp
1½ cups diced cooked crab-meat
1 cup cut-up canned asparagus spears

1 cup sliced celery
1 cup cooked peas
1 small head of lettuce, shred-ded

Dressing

1 clove garlic
4 tablespoons good vinegar
8 tablespoons salad oil

1¼ teaspoons salt
1 teaspoon paprika
Freshly ground pepper

Garnish

2 hard-cooked eggs, sliced

3 tomatoes, peeled and sliced

Clean mushrooms; slice lengthwise. Sprinkle with few drops lemon juice. Keep in covered bowl in refrigerator. Peel shrimp. Leave whole, or cut lengthwise. Keep crabmeat and shrimp in refrigerator until serving time. Make dressing: Place all ingredients in a jar; cover, and shake until blended.

Half an hour before serving, assemble all salad ingredients; arrange in layers in salad bowl that has been rubbed with garlic. Pour dressing over salad, and toss lightly. Garnish with rows of egg and tomato slices. Chill before serving. (Salad can also be served from a large platter, with a few lettuce leaves in the center and salad piled high on lettuce. Arrange garnish in rows around salad.) Makes 5 or 6 servings.

TOMATO RING
Tomatring
(Traditional)

3 large onions
2 pounds tomatoes (8 medium)
10½-ounce can consomme
2 teaspoons salt
2 teaspoons sugar
1/8 teaspoon pepper
2 envelopes unflavored gelatin

¼ cup cold water
1 tablespoon butter or margarine
1 tablespoon flour
¼ cup heavy cream, whipped
Watercress

Peel and slice onions and tomatoes. Place in saucepan with consomme and seasonings. Bring to boil; lower heat, and cook until vegetables are tender. Force through fine sieve.

Sprinkle gelatin on cold water; let stand a few minutes. Melt butter in saucepan. Add flour, and stir until blended. Gradually add tomato puree; cook, stirring, until smooth. Add gelatin mixture. Brush oil on ring mold, and pour in gelatin mixture. Chill until firm. Loosen gelatin ring, and turn onto serving dish. Garnish with whipped cream and watercress. Serve with slices of boiled ham, as part of smorgasbord or as luncheon dish. Makes 6 servings.

SWEDISH ROAST PORK
Ugnstekt Kotlettrad
(Traditional)

3½-pound round loin of pork (backbone removed)
1 teaspoon salt
1½ teaspoons powdered ginger

¼ teaspoon black pepper
⅓ teaspoon dried sage

Preheat oven to 350°. Combine salt, ginger, pepper, and sage, and rub into pork. Place pork in shallow roasting pan, fat side up. Roast 1½ hours. Makes 6 to 8 servings.

DIET SWEDISH ROAST PORK

Prepare in traditional way, but drain and blot all fat.

GLAZED SWEDISH CHRISTMAS HAM
Kokt Griljerad Skinka
(Traditional)

6-pound canned ham
Pinch marjoram
Dash rosemary
2 eggs (or 2 egg whites)
¼ cup prepared mustard
2 tablespoons brown sugar

¼ cup finely ground dry bread
  crumbs
½ cup water
¼ cup crab-apple jelly
½ cup golden raisins

Preheat oven to 325°. Place ham, fat side down, in baking pan with gelatin from can; bake 1 hour. Remove from oven. Set oven to 400°. Combine eggs (or egg whites), mustard, and sugar. Turn ham fat side up, and spread with egg mixture, using a pastry brush. Sprinkle evenly with bread crumbs. Return ham to oven; bake until crumbs are browned—approximately 10 minutes. Remove from oven, and place on a large serving platter or carving board for about 10 minutes, to seal in the juices. Meanwhile, add water to the baking pan; loosen crusty pieces at bottom of pan, and bring water to a boil. Strain into a small, heavy, enamel-clad saucepan. Add jelly and raisins, and heat, stirring as the jelly dissolves. Serve jelly sauce hot over hot or cold ham slices. Serve with Spiced Red Cabbage, below. Makes 10-12 servings.

DIET GLAZED SWEDISH CHRISTMAS HAM

Prepare traditional recipe, with the following exceptions: Use sugar substitute to equal 2 tablespoons brown sugar and dietetic jelly.

SPICED RED CABBAGE
Kokt Rodkal
(Traditional)

3 tablespoons safflower margarine or butter
6 cups shredded red cabbage
2 cups cored, peeled, and sliced apples
2 tablespoons maple syrup or molasses
1 cup minced onion
1/3 cup red-wine vinegar

2 teaspoons crushed caraway seeds
1 cup water
1 teaspoon salt
1/8 teaspoon savory
Dash tarragon
2 tablespoons red-currant jelly
2 teaspoons orange juice

Melt margarine in large, heavy skillet or saucepan. Add cabbage, apples, and syrup; cover, and bring to a boil, stirring once or twice to blend. Lower heat, and add remaining ingredients. Cover, and simmer about 45 minutes, or until cabbage and apples are tender. Add more water if needed. Remove cover during last 10 minutes, so excess liquid will evaporate. Serve with Glazed Swedish Christmas Ham. Makes 10-12 servings.

DIET SPICED RED CABBAGE

Prepare traditional recipe, but substitute diet margarine for safflower margarine or butter and diet syrup for maple syrup.

SMALL MEATBALLS
Sma Kottbullar
(Traditional)

¼ cup finely chopped onion
1 tablespoon shortening
¼ cup fine dry bread crumbs
⅓ cup water
⅓ cup cream
1 pound lean ground sirloin
¼ pound lean ground pork
2 tablespoons salt

¼ teaspoon pepper
1/8 teaspoon rosemary
1/8 teaspoon cloves
⅓ cup butter or safflower margarine
¼ cup boiling water
1 tablespoon cornstarch

Saute onion in shortening until transparent and golden. Soak crumbs in mixture of ⅓ cups water and cream. Combine onion, crumb mixture, meats, seasonings, and herbs; mix thoroughly until smooth. Wet your hands, to keep the mixture from sticking, and shape it into small balls with your palms. Fry in butter until evenly brown. Shake the pan constantly, to keep the meatballs rounded. When all meatballs are browned, reduce heat to low; cover pan, and simmer 8 minutes (15 minutes for larger meatballs). Remove meatballs; pour off fat. Add boiling water to cornstarch to blend. Add to the pan; stir over moderate heat until mixture comes to a boil. Add seasoning to taste. Serve gravy with meatballs. Makes about 35 small meatballs.

DIET SMALL MEATBALLS

Use traditional recipe, but omit gravy.

BRAISED VEAL BIRDS
Kalvrullader
(Traditional)

1½ pounds (8 slices) veal escalops, cut 3/8 inch thick
¼ cup unbleached flower
¼ teaspoon salt
¼ teaspoon white pepper
8 thin slices boiled ham, 3-by-7 inches

8 thin slices Swiss cheese, 3-by-7 inches
2 tablespoons safflower salad oil
½ cup beef bouillon
Pinch marjoram
¼ cup whole milk (or cream)

Pound meat with mallet to ¼-inch thickness; then trim into 4-by-8-inch rectangles. Mix flour and seasonings in shallow dish. Coat meat on both sides. Place a slice of ham and a slice of cheese on each meat slice. Roll up lengthwise, and fasten with toothpicks. Heat oil in heavy iron or aluminum skillet. Add meat; brown quickly on both sides. Add hot beef bouillon with a pinch of marjoram; cover tightly, and simmer ½ hour. Lift veal birds out of pan and into a deep serving dish. Add milk to liquid in skillet, and cook 2 minutes. Remove toothpicks from veal birds. Pour gravy over birds. Garnish with parsley, and serve. Makes 6 servings.

DIET BRAISED VEAL BIRDS

1½ pounds (8 slices) veal escalops, cut 3/8 inch thick
4 ounces ground veal
1 cup chopped celery
1 cup minced onion (or the dehydrated equivalent)
1 cup chopped mushrooms (fresh or canned)

Salt, white pepper, garlic and onion powder to taste
Skimmed milk
8 thin slices boiled ham
3 cups beef bouillon
Paprika
16 pearl onions
8 sprigs parsley

Pound meat with mallet to ¼-inch thickness; trim into 4-by-8-inch rectangles. Prepare filling: Mix ground veal, celery, minced onion, half the mushrooms, and the seasonings. Add a little skimmed milk to hold mixture together. Arrange veal escalops in a row, and place a slice of ham on each. Separate filling into 8 equal portions, and place on ham. Roll up each veal slice, and fasten with toothpicks or tie with white string. Broil, 3 to 4 inches from heat, just enough to brown lightly on both sides. Turn once. Place beef bouillon in heavy iron or aluminum skillet, and bring to a boil. Place veal birds in the bouillon so they are just half covered. Sprinkle with paprika. Cover tightly; turn heat to medium, and simmer 10 minutes. Add pearl onions; simmer 10 minutes more, or until veal birds are tender. Lift birds out of skillet, and arrange in deep serving dish. Add remaining mushrooms to liquid in skillet; stir once, and pour over meat, as a sauce. Garnish each serving with parsley. Makes 6 servings.

CRUSTY LAMB ROAST

4 pounds boned and rolled leg
of lamb
½ cup mustard
¼ cup Diet Lingonberry Jam
1 tablespoon soy sauce
½ teaspoon onion salt
¼ teaspoon garlic powder

2 tablespoons minced de-
hydrated onion
½ teaspoon crushed rosemary
Pinch marjoram
1 tablespoon sesame or safflower oil

Remove lamb from refrigerator ½ hour before cooking. Preheat
oven to 350°. Prepare crust: Place mustard and jam in a glass
bowl. Stir in all seasonings except oil. After 3 minutes, to allow
softening of dehydrated onion and herbs, beat mixture with wire
whisk. Continue beating as you add the oil, drop by drop, until
mixture thickens. Place lamb on rack in roasting pan; coat with
crust mixture. Roast just below center of the oven for 1 hour and
45 minutes. (Reduce roasting time 15 minutes if you prefer lamb
European style, pink and juicy.) Remove from oven, and let stand
15 minutes to ½ hour before carving and serving. Makes 10-12
servings.

SWEDISH CHEESECAKE
Smalandskostkaka
(Traditional)

¾ cup chopped toasted
  almonds
3 eggs
1 teaspoon lemon juice
¼ cup sugar

2 cups light cream
½ teaspoon almond extract
¼ cup cake flour
2⅓ cups cottage cheese

Preheat oven to 350°. Toast almonds slightly, and chop coarsely. (Do not chop to powder.) Place eggs, lemon juice, sugar, cream and almond extract in a mixing bowl, and beat with electric or manual mixer until eggs are thoroughly mixed with cream. Combine flour and ½ cup of the almonds, and slowly add egg mixture, beating all the while. Add cheese, and mix well. Pour into well-greased 8-inch or 9-inch fluted pie pan; sprinkle with remaining almonds, and bake approximately 1 hour, until inserted knife comes out clean. Cool, then chill. Serve topped with whipped cream and berries in season, or with jelly. Makes 6-8 servings.

DIET SWEDISH CHEESECAKE

¾ cup chopped toasted
  almonds
3 eggs
1 tablespoon lemon juice
2½ teaspoons melted diet
  margarine
Granulated-sugar substitute
  equal to ¼ cup sugar

1 teaspoon vanilla extract
½ teaspoon almond extract
1 tablespoon cornstarch
2⅓ cups ricotta or skimmed
  milk cottage cheese

Preheat oven to 350°. Toast almonds slightly, and chop coarsely. Place ½ cup of the almonds and all other ingredients, except cheese, in a mixing bowl, and whip thoroughly with electric or manual mixer. Add cheese, and mix until smooth. Pour into non-stick or lecithin-sprayed loaf pan, to keep cheesecake from falling; sprinkle with remaining almonds, and bake 45 minutes. Open oven door; let cheesecake remain in oven 1 hour. Remove, cool, and refrigerate until chilled, or overnight. Makes 6-8 servings.

ALMOND-FILLED BAKED APPLES
Mandelfyllda Stekta Applen
(Traditional)

4 egg whites
½ cup water
½ cup sugar
½ teaspoon almond extract
2 cups blanched and ground
  almonds

6 large baking apples
3 tablespoons melted butter or
  margarine
1 cup dry bread crumbs

Puree egg whites, water, sugar, almond extract, and almonds in blender 30 seconds, or until ingredients are of paste consistency. Core and peel apples, leaving 1 or 2 inches of skin at their base. Brush apples with butter; then roll in bread crumbs. Arrange in shallow baking dish with 1/8 inch of water. Spoon almond filling into centers of apples. Combine remaining crumbs, butter, and almond filling to cap the apples. Bake at 350° for 1 hour. Serve topped with Diet Lemon-Custard Sauce. Makes 6 servings.

DIET ALMOND-FILLED BAKED APPLES

Follow traditional recipe, with these substitutions: granulated-sugar substitute equivalent to ½ cup sugar, diet margarine, Granola-type cereal instead of almonds.

DIET LEMON-CUSTARD SAUCE

4 eggs

Liquid sugar substitute equal to
4 teaspoons sugar

½ teaspoon lemon extract

¼ teaspoon imitation butter
flavoring

2 cups water

⅔ cup skimmed-milk powder

1/8 teaspoon almond extract

Beat eggs to fluff. Combine sugar substitute, lemon extract, and butter flavoring with eggs; mix well. Spray double-boiler top with lecithin coating. Pour water into top of boiler; add skimmed-milk powder slowly, stirring to dissolve. Heat over boiling water until milk mixture is very hot, but not boiling. Remove double-boiler top from heat. Add egg mixture slowly, stirring all the while. Return to bottom of double boiler, and heat only until sauce thickens. Add almond extract. Use sauce hot or cold over baked apples.

PART VI
MAKING YOUR MIND
WORK FOR YOU

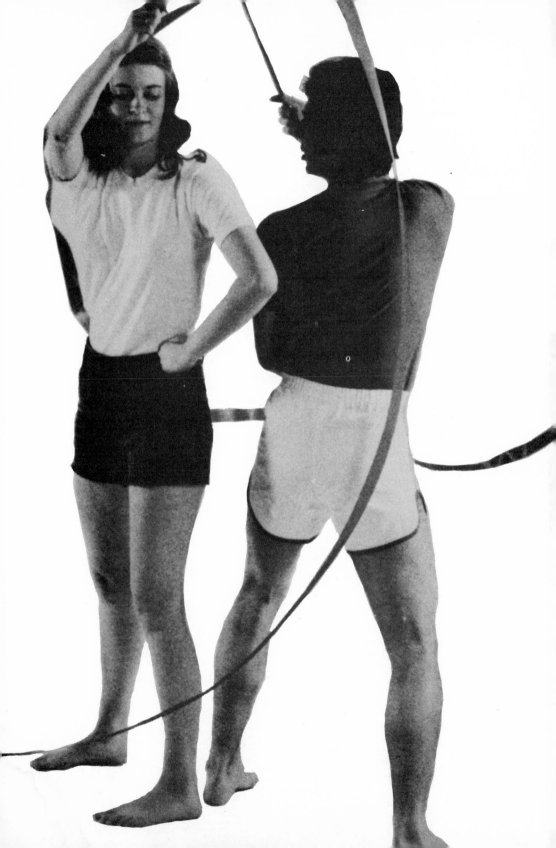

TWELVE

THE MAGIC OF YOUR MIND

The mind has its own magic. Every drama has its plot. Every city has its plan. Every project has its goal.

And every life has its design, controlled by the magic of your mind.

The zest of the Swedish people for living is exhilarating and contagious. They refuse to play Russian roulette with their lives. Good health and long life are not fearfully pursued goals but joyous daily involvements.

We are born, it is hoped, with a sound heart, a working circulatory system, and sound plumbing. We have but one life, and for this one life we are given two options: we may prolong life by establishing and nurturing positive, optimistic, healthy attitudes, values. Or we may shorten it by accepting the slow, insidious destruction of fear, hatreds, small thinking, pettiness, and by the failure to exercise our bodies and our minds in reaching for bold, worthwhile objectives.

The design needn't be all structured and detailed like a meticulous blueprint. The design for living can be opening your heart to the world. . . . Giving without anticipating and getting. . . . Keeping all your senses alive, so that you don't miss the beauty of a sunset, the charm of a baby's smile, the fragrance of a new-mown field, the thrill of bird song, the delicate loveliness of snow on slender branches. . . . Making your commitment, deciding and enjoying the struggle entailed in what you stand for. . . . Sustaining the element of hope, joy, positiveness.

As you master control over your thoughts, clarify healthy thinking-patterns, translate dreams to action that rewards you with small, then increasingly significant achievements, you experience the heady gratification of self-discovery. How marvelous to learn that your potential is far greater than you once imagined! To discover your very worthiness and your range of powers to appreciate, to encourage and inspire others, to understand, to attain new knowledge and acquire new skills and talents and aptitudes!

All these treasures can be made yours by touching your own life with the magic wand of your own mental powers.

There are many more wonders that can be brought about, more gratifications that can be made yours by the phenomenal powers in your own mind. They may come in the small hours of the night when the crickets' calls and the automobiles' wheel sounds fall into silence. Then you may discover the rich comfort of silence, the soft, pleasant feeling of delicious isolation from outside forces, when you can feel at one with something larger than your customary daily contacts and experience a quiet sense of serenity and receptivity of fresh ideas, new and more wonderful dreams you can help come true.

For contrast, give your mind the freedom to help you escape from loneliness, for it can be a wonderful companion of itself and a guide to even more delightful companions. Let it lead you to the library, guide your hand to the books and periodicals that teach you those things you always wanted to learn, bring you the friendship of stimulating authors through their works, show you new directions for thought, learning, action, and involvement. There can never be loneliness for someone who has the capacity to reject boredom as unworthy of a vigorous, creative mind. In your pursuit of activities you find rewarding, you may well join with others in classrooms, organizations, research projects, friendly discussions, and such outside-yourself pursuits readily supplant loneliness with companionship and growth you will enjoy.

Always through bringing joy to others do we gain the greatest gratifications for ourselves. Who can you help who is worthy of such assistance? What talents, understanding, patience, companionship have you to give? Guidance for the troubled young? Reading for the blind? Transportation for the handicapped? Time and attention for the old? The needs are there, all around us, and, in giving of ourselves to fill those needs, we may derive unbelievable fulfillments for ourselves.

Get outdoors! Let nature talk to you, caress you, teach you! Watch delicate, pale-green young leaves timidly thrust from the twigs, grow, strengthen, feed the sun's nourishment to the host plant, and feel the parallel in yourself. Experience the intoxicating glory of a sunrise; know that the day it's bringing you is your day, a day of achievement and of sharing and giving and the joys those actions bring. See the flowers in their beauty, and wonder about other beauty around you that is equally generous in sharing its color and fragrance and charm with you. Listen to water. Feel the sun's warmth. Belong in this superlative, ever-changing kaleidoscope of the senses that is nature, and let your mind bask in the wonder of it all.

Then, when you focus that marvel of your mind on people problems, many of them become much easier to solve. Maybe it was just attention they wanted. Perhaps it was an inadvertent thing that caused the tension, a misunderstanding. Look for the good in others. Find their motivations. Get your thoughts away from yourself and directed to them with charity, kindness, and understanding. You can never hate someone you really understand, into whose skin and thoughts you have let yourself penetrate so that you can see from his or her viewpoint.

Enjoy the realization that you are someone special, unique, blessed with countless powers, numerous capabilities. It's easy to like someone with the understanding, the insight, the selflessness, and still the self-realization that you possess.

Unlimber that mind of yours. When you awaken in the morning, enjoy the expectancy of what this glorious day will bring. Be alert to discovery, an interesting doorway, a phase of a companion you hadn't appreciated or known about before, a good quality in yourself you hadn't identified previously. The sense of expectancy is important magic for that mind of yours, and it can be a bearer of much joy.

Don't let others define what is success for you. Set your own standards, your own goals. Too often the success cult breeds destruction and unhappiness when it is measured by costly possessions, tawdry achievements, formidable titles, or difficult-to-keep-up symbols. What do you really want for yourself, not to impress or mollify others? Success comes from achieving these goals, not those imposed on you by others.

Every individual must set his own self-objectives, the special wishes he hopes to grant himself by the magic of his mind.

We rather like those objectives we associate with the many people with whom it was our privilege to work in researching and distilling the principles of the Royal Swedish Way To Keep Fit:

The creation of love and friendship.

The gift of love.

The recognition and enjoyment of happiness.

APPENDICES

We are often tempted to think that because we are exercising we can eat more of those foods considered fattening than we can when not exercising. And that is true, but only up to a point. To keep you from going overboard on favorite foods, run your eye down the figures on this page. They tell you how many calories you are using during your daily activities.

DAILY ACTIVITY	CALORIES YOU WILL USE PER DAY FOR EACH ONE POUND OF WEIGHT	
	MEN	WOMEN
Studying	16	15
Editing	16	15
Typing	18	19
Playing a musical instrument	18	19
Bookkeeping	18	19
Selling	20	21
Painting	20	21
Serving table	20	21
Farming	23	25
Housecleaning	23	25
House painting	23	25
Moving furniture	36	36
Road building	36	36
Stone working	36	36

244

IF YOUR CHILDREN WANT TO DIET

The United States Department of Health, Education and Welfare has prepared a list of foods that will meet the needs of healthy children from the ages of one to six. If your youngsters want to (or should be) on a diet, take the USDA recommendations into consideration in planning diets for them, and discuss the diet you propose with your pediatrician or family doctor.

FOOD	DAILY REQUIREMENT	PORTION FOR	
		2-3 YEARS	4-5 YEAR
Milk	3-4 cups	1/2-1 cup	1 cup
Citrus fruits for Vitamin C	1 medium orange or 1/3 cup citrus or 2/3 cup tomato juice	1/3-1/2 cup	1/3-1/2 cup
Eggs	1	1	1
Butter or fortified margarine	Spread thinly on bread, used sparingly on vegetables		
Cereal; whole grain, enriched or restored	1 serving	1/2 cup	1/2 cup
Bread, whole grain or enriched	1 1/2-3 slices	1 slice	1 1/2 slices
Meat, poultry, fish cottage cheese	1-4 tbsp.	2-3 tbsp.	4 tbsp.
Potatoes, white or sweet	1 serving	3 tbsp.	4 tbsp.
Cooked vegetables, leafy deep green or yellow	1-2 servings	3 tbsp.	3-4 tbsp.
Raw vegetables	1 serving		
Fruits other than citrus	1 serving	1/3 cup	1/2 cup

IF YOUR TEENAGERS WANT TO DIET

With your doctor's permission, they can follow adult diet plans. However, be aware that teenagers have a unique metabolism, one we are still learning more about, and which appears to have characteristics distinctly different from an adult's. During the teen years, leafy green and yellow vegetables are essential, and so is milk (though sodas may be more fun). Vitamin A is a promoter of a glowing complexion and is considered essential in maintaining good vision. Also, see to it that your teenagers get lots of citrus fruits, tomatoes and raw cabbage, which are the vegetables and fruits associated with vitamin C. If they argue, tell them those vegetables keep their energy levels high. For teenagers, a daily diet that includes four or more servings of foods containing vitamins A and C is recommended.

The New Jersey Department of Health in 1960 issued a diet manual describing foods permitted, and those not permitted, for people avoiding cholesterol. Here's a capsule of that information:

FOODS	PERMITTED	AVOIDED
Soups	Clear soups and vegetable soups with all fat removed.	Cream soups, meat soups and others with fat
Meat, Fish, Poultry	Lean meats and poultry with skin removed. White fish such as flounder, haddock, cod.	Liver, brains, and other organ meats; bacon; shellfish, seafood, and fish roe; duck, goose; packaged luncheon meats, hot dogs.
Vegetables	All except those noted in next column (potatoes are fine).	Your physician may recommend you avoid the cabbagy vegetables, such as broccoli, cauliflower, brussels sprouts; cucumbers; turnips; onions; radishes; dried peas, beans and lentils.
Starches	Rice, macaroni, noodles, spaghetti; whole grain or enriched bread and cereals; graham crackers; saltines.	Cocktail crackers containing fats; pancakes, waffles, doughnuts and other fried or fatty pastries.
Dairy Products	Skim milk cheese, Egg whites; skim milk or skimmed-milk dairy products.	Avoid all others: Whole milk and all whole-milk dairy products.
Sweets	Gelatin desserts, and prepared desserts made with skim milk; angel food cake; jelly, honey, sugar, jams, preserves; candies (such as hard candy) made from sugar.	All desserts, including pastries containing egg yolk, butter, whole milk, or whole-milk products such as cream cheese and cream; puddings containing fats or whole milk; ice creams containing cream or whole milk; chocolate and chocolate products; nuts.

Fruits	All fruits; frozen, canned, fresh.	None restricted.
Drinks	Tea; coffee; herb teas.	Alcohols are restricted, and drinks containing alcohol.
Fats	Vegetable oils and salad dressings with vegetable oils.	Dairy and meat fat products, such as butter, cream, lard, bacon fat, chicken and other poultry fats, and solidified vegetable shortening including margarine. Foods fried in fats other than vegetable fats.

This list cannot be considered a replacement for a doctor's advice on the subject of foods permitted those with cholesterol difficulties. If you have a cholesterol problem, or suspect you may have one, have a thorough check-up and discuss any proposed diet plans with your family doctor.

DIET DICTIONARY

FOODS HIGH IN PROTEINS

Milk	Poultry
Skim milk	Fish
Buttermilk	Soybeans
Evaporated milk	Nuts
Condensed milk	Peanut butter
Cheese	Beans (dried)
Eggs	Lentils (dried)
Liver	Peas (dried)
Kidney	Cereals
Meats (all types)	Whole grain flour

FOODS HIGH IN FATS

Chocolate	Pork products
Ice cream	Liver
Cream	Egg yolks
Whole milk	Vegetable oil
Sour cream	Custard and pie fillings
Butter	Cheese
Margarine	Fatty meats
Meat fats	

FOODS HIGH IN CARBOHYDRATES

Sugar	Cereals	Beans
Candy	Breads	Peas
Chocolate	Rolls	Lentils
Syrups	Macaroni	Fruits (all types)
Jellies	Noodles	Sodas
Jams	Cakes	
Preserves	Pies	
Honey	Crackers	
Flour	Rice	
Spaghetti	Cornstarch	

DIET DICTIONARY

FOODS HIGH IN VITAMIN A

Yellow vegetables
Green vegetables
Yellow cheese
Whole milk
Liver
Cantaloupe
Carrots
Broccoli
Sweet potatoes

Peas
Spinach
Peaches
Tomatoes
Corn
Apricots
Butter
Margarine

FOODS HIGH IN VITAMIN C

Oranges
Lemons
Limes
Grapefruits
Tomatoes
Leafy greens
Strawberries

Cabbage
Potatoes, white
Green peppers
Red peppers
Pineapples
Sweet potatoes

THE LONGEVITY TEST

More and more recognition is being given by psychologists to emotion that can decrease longevity. Below are thirty questions relating to life-terminating emotions: impatience, frustration, hate, envy, jealousy, anxiety, avarice. The purpose of the test is to raise your consciousness of damaging emotions. The results of this test follow.

1. Do you dread waking up in the morning?
2. Are you often late for work/school? Dates?
3. Do you often fail to get everything done during the day?
4. Do you begrudge sharing the attention of your friends?
5. Are you resentful at work/school?
6. Are your comments about others often disparaging?

7. Does anyone in your close entourage irritate you maddeningly?
8. Do you criticize as many as four in ten people you pass in the street?
9. Are you deeply envious of others?
10. Do you tend to blame others for your lack of success?
11. Do you resent the wealth or health of a relative or close friend?
12. Do you feel that others patronize you?
13. Do you feel inferior to well-dressed people?
14. Do you consider yourself physically unattractive?
15. Do you blame yourself when others are moody?
16. Do you daydream about owning the possessions of others?
17. Are you susceptible to minor illnesses?
18. Do you feel belittled in the presence of attractive people?
19. Do you tire easily?
20. Do you spend too much on non-essentials to raise your spirits?
21. Are you afraid to express your real feelings?
22. Do you lack self-confidence?
23. Are you very timid or shy?
24. Do you have many vague aches or pains?
25. Do you worry about how you impress others?
26. Do you procrastinate?
27. Do you resent being teased by a good friend?
28. Does any failure leave you feeling unworthy?
29. Do you suspect your closest friends don't really care?
30. Are you obsessed about people you dislike?

A "yes" to any to these suggests you may be allowing a life-terminating emotion into your mind, but the truth is only highly disciplined people can keep them all out. A vigorous exercise program can dissipate some of the effects of the stresses these emotions create. Since mental and physical health are symbiotic, or closely related, almost any exercise program that gets the blood going is likely to leave you feeling better mentally and help you control negative, life-terminating emotions.
To rate your score:
If you answered "yes" to up to five questions, your mental health is great.

If you answered "yes" to between five and ten questions, your mental health is good.

If you answered "yes" to between ten and fifteen questions, your mental health is average.

If you answered "yes" to between fifteen and twenty questions, your mental health is poor.

If you answered "yes" to more than twenty questions, your mental health needs serious attention.